The International Library

MAN'S UNCONSCIOUS
PASSION

Founded by C. K. Ogden

The International Library of Psychology

GENERAL PSYCHOLOGY
In 38 Volumes

MAN'S UNCONSCIOUS PASSION

WILFRID LAY

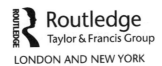

Routledge
Taylor & Francis Group

LONDON AND NEW YORK

First published in 1921 by
Kegan Paul, Trench, Trubner & Co., Ltd.
2 Park Square, Milton Park, Abingdon, Oxfordshire OX14 4RN
711 Third Avenue, New York, NY 10017

First issued in paperback 2014

Routledge is an imprint of the Taylor and Francis Group, an informa business

British Library Cataloguing in Publication Data
A CIP catalogue record for this book
is available from the British Library

Man's Unconscious Passion
ISBN 978-0415-21031-7
General Psychology: 38 Volumes
ISBN 0415-21129-8
The International Library of Psychology: 204 Volumes
ISBN 0415-19132-7

ISBN 13: 978-1-138-87532-6 (pbk)
ISBN 13: 978-0-415-21031-7 (hbk)

TABLE OF CONTENTS

v

CONTENTS

MAN'S UNCONSCIOUS PASSION

MAN'S UNCONSCIOUS PASSION

CHAPTER I

THE TOTAL SITUATION

A. *Influence*

SOME infinitesimal influence is exerted by you on everything else in the universe, if only from the fact that you occupy space. And some influence is exerted upon you by every other thing in space, a greater influence from the things of your environment, a still greater from the immediate environment. But what is the environment? It is safe to say that unless there were some interrelation of cause and effect between the individual and his environment, there would be no significance in its being called an environment. The things that cause changes in your mental and physical behaviour are your environment, and the more effect they have, the more are you environed by them.

It would be difficult to say by what you are most influenced. Some might think that it was by your physical surroundings, some by your

1

heredity. The most catholic will see that you
are the net result of all the causes, physical and
mental, that have operated on you from the beginning of time, and that there are many elements entering into the total situation that could
be called causative of it, but that are not apparent to your consciousness, although undoubtedly they do make impressions upon your sense
organs.

The total situation for the unconscious is
always much more extensive than it is for consciousness. Outside of conscious hearing there
are sound waves continually impinging upon the
ear-drum, and, whether or not they are in the
form of spoken words, they will have an influence upon the psyche, even if they never enter
consciousness. In the realm of sight there are
impressions that never enter consciousness at
all, however much they may be making vibra-
tions in the rods and cones of the retina. In
touch you have constant skin pressures of which
you are rarely conscious, though you may from
time to time become aware of them.

In general, the impressions that are constantly
being made upon all the sense organs, external
and internal, are the total situation in which, at
any given time, you are involved; and only a
very small number of these are illuminated by
the searchlight of consciousness, as it turns now

in one direction (to one sense quality) and now in another.

But however narrow is the scope of consciousness itself, and however few of the elements of this total situation it illuminates for your mental gaze, to speak figuratively, the total situation, consisting of all the impressions from without, whether in consciousness or not, and of all the impressions from within (organic sensations), and of all the ideas, verbal, and otherwise sensory, both conscious and unconscious,— this total situation is always perceptible to the unconscious mind. Your behaviour is never determined by what is in consciousness alone. The total situation as I have called it, you have always with you. No part of it is without influence upon your behaviour, physical and mental. Your physical behaviour is partly visible to your eyes, and otherwise consciously perceptible to other senses, but only a small proportion of it. Similarly your mental behaviour, which is the ideas, feelings, images, emotions, wishes, desires, volitions, etc., or whatever else you include by the terms usually applied to mental phenomena, your total mental behaviour is almost entirely outside of that circle of conscious illumination referred to above.

No definite idea can be gained by the observer concerning the actual shape of an iceberg *below the surface* of the water, but, whatever shape it may be, we know that it is from eight to nine times as great in volume as what appears above the surface. Whatever then may be in our consciousness at any time, we may be quite sure that a great deal more is in our mind but not in our consciousness. If a sphere of wood, a hundred feet in diameter, were in the water, and its specific gravity were 90%, one-tenth of it would be above the surface. If it were a perfect sphere of homogeneous density throughout, it could be rotated on any axis by the slightest touch of a finger, and any part of its surface could be brought into view above the level of the water.

But, to carry out this metaphor, the mind is neither spherical, nor is it of homogeneous density throughout. Possibly the iceberg is the best illustration of the extent of the conscious and unconscious mind, because it is irregular in shape, may be melted off at the bottom by warm currents, and lean over or turn turtle according to circumstances. The work of psychoanalysis is to make the thing spherical, so to speak, in order that it may be turned over and examined on every side. If one attempted to overturn a large, flat piece of ice in the water one would have to lift a goodly proportion of its weight.

The whole iceberg in this figure represents the total situation. Most of the total situation is imperceptible to consciousness, but to the mental elaboration of what enters consciousness, it is the amount of ice under the water necessary to raise the rest of it above the surface. There would not be so much above, if there were less underneath. The centre of gravity of the whole mass determines the part of the iceberg that shall appear above the water's surface. Every part that appears, does so because of the weight and shape of the whole.

Exactly the same may be said of the conscious elements of the total mental situation, so much of which is unconscious. The most active and aggressive men are so because of the greatness of their unconscious desires. What appears on the surface of their conduct, both words and actions, is largely, if not totally, determined by what is beneath. We do not see what is beneath; we merely deduce the existence of it, but the deduction is quite as valid as that for the existence of other consciousness besides our own.

B. *The Unconscious Deducible*

That another person has a consciousness like mine is deduction only, not experience. That my own mind is part unconscious is similarly deducible and with exactly the same logic. My own unconscious is to me as little a matter of

direct perception as is to me the consciousness
of a person other than myself. I infer both, and
with absolutely equal validity. Never do I doubt
for a minute that others have consciousness as
I have. Never should I doubt that my mind has
means of modifying, as it has means of storing,
my experiences and other expressions. I see the
acts of others, and make my own inferences as
to what caused these acts. I see my own acts
and should make the same kind of inferences as
to what caused them. I can see perfectly that
what Brown really admires about Miss Green is
her money, and not her character or her person.
I can see clearly how he is deceiving himself.
But I never make the same inference about myself—that I am deceiving myself about the true
motives of any wooing or doing of my own. In
order fully to know myself I should have to
make the same inferences about myself that I
make about others.

C. *Unconscious and Foreconscious*

It must not be supposed that there is a sharp
line of demarkation between consciousness and
the unconscious, but that certain mental activities can be brought at once and with little effort into full consciousness, while others can
never be brought into clear consciousness at all,

for one reason, possibly, that they are not expressible in the ordinary medium of verbal, pictorial or other sensory-motor means of expression, possibly because the effort would be too great to have any value. The results would either be unrecognizable or would be worth little or nothing.

But between the mental activities that are so unconscious, so inaccessible, and so unavailable for conscious presentation, and the mental activities that pop into, and out of, consciousness spontaneously or accompanied by a feeling of volition, there is an endless series of gradations. To that degree of difficulty of resuscitation shown by the multiplication table, the Lord's Prayer and sundry prices, street and telephone numbers, some writers give the name *Foreconscious*. The mental activities labelled with this name are comparatively easy to evoke, and they are accompanied by a more vividly pleasant sense of effort than are the attempts to evoke the activities that generally take place in the lower strata of the truly and inexorably unconscious.

There is no doubt, however, that a great many of the complexes and other difficulties, irregularities of functioning and mild mental disorders are connected with activities of the so-called foreconscious level.

Another important consideration must not be

overlooked that distinguishes foreconscious activities from the truly unconscious kind.

The foreconscious mental processes are presentable, that is, available for ready revivification or illumination, by virtue of their being unopposed by the influences of society which works upon and through the upper, more conscious, levels of the mind. By more conscious here, is meant more presentable. The more presentable are those which find less opposition from the influences exerted through the upper levels, and thus come into consciousness more frequently and more clearly than those against which society has raised obstructions.

Thus there struggle up toward expression in the higher mental levels, vague, amorphous cravings for activity, for warmth and light, and for mere assertiveness and aggrandizement of the ego. These take definite form from the individual's perception of things in the external world. The infant having been contented with aimlessly exercising its muscles, the child now begins to realize the difference between himself and the external world, and, if left to himself, would first grasp and gather around him, everything from which came pleasant sensations, and would push away everything unpleasant; and second, would expend his energy on the things found pleasant until, by destroying them, he found them unpleasant. By this extension of his physical activity, he expands his objective ego and thus satisfies his indefinite craving for aggrandizement.

But about this time he becomes aware of the similar tendency of the other personalities to enlarge themselves. This tumescent tendency, if left to itself, would result in the greater or stronger of two individuals annhilating the lesser or weaker. Then first enters the embryo concept of concerted action, in which even two children will work together and make a pile of pleasant things greater than the sum of the two separate piles. Then the social instinct comes into play, which is the basis of all later team work, organized effort and community work of every sort. Here the objects of the previously exceedingly indefinite craving become more and more definite desires. In other words, the desire becomes loosely attached to definite objects and experiences, always presupposing that they fulfil the requirements of the still existing powerful craving for activity, aggrandizement, warmth and light. It is not to be doubted that the search for the North Pole was ultimately based on a craving for the warmth and light of public appreciation, no matter how cold and dark the actual experiences may have been.

The more definite the objects to which desire is attached, the more numerous are the individuals who desire the same thing. This leads to the necessary conflict between two individuals desiring the same; and an ultimate compromise, a division of the thing into parts, either spatially or temporally. A cake or an apple or an estate can be divided, a chair can be used by two persons in turn. This works very well until the still more developed individual is not satisfied with communal possession, but only with possession containing the element of exclusiveness. Then the parts of the objective ego, be they chairs or estates, must be carefully kept for exclusive use. No one else may use them, even when the person, of whose external ego they form a part, is not using them, a feeling probably due to the feeling of unpleasantness experienced in finding another sitting in one's chair or occupying one's estate, and in getting him to vacate. The unpleasantness of this feeling is in turn largely determined by an unconscious feeling that the other fellow really has as much right to it morally as oneself.

That the number of individuals desiring the same thing is increased by the definiteness of desires arises from the innateness of imitation. Imitation in turn comes from the interrelation of sensory and motor processes in the body. For example, I reproduce in my own body, minute muscular contractions, when I see others moving, as in walking, dancing, playing ball. These minute contractions are made in me reflexly, automatically, and are a transmuted visual sensation. That is, they are transmuted from a visual impression into a movement, or innervation of muscles, very minute, but which, if carried out in large, would constitute the same motions in me that are being made by the person at whom I am looking. This is true not only of movements but of positions of the body, when it is not moving. Seeing a person sitting makes me unconsciously, for a moment at least, imagine myself as sitting. This means that it causes a nerve impulse tending to produce the sitting posture, to be sent to the muscles which would put me or hold me in the sitting posture looked at. Seeing a person yawn produces in me the same imitative unconscious tendency. So does seeing a person laugh make me laugh, although I may not know what he is laughing about. Thus it is clear that unconscious imitation of the acts of others goes on in us all the time. In children it is quite noticeable.

Reflex, unconscious, minute imitation is an important psychical as well as physical fact. It is true, too, not only of the contractions of the larger so-called voluntary muscles, but also of those of the smaller involuntary muscles controlling the calibre of various vessels in the body and the working of various glands that produce both internal and external secretions.

But in the working of the smaller vessels and glands, a great part is played by ideas. It should not be forgotten that an idea has many forms in the mind. The same idea may have a visual form, an auditory form, a gustatory form, an olfactory form, a tactual form, a muscular form, or a form consisting of organic or any other kind of images. It may be difficult to accept the fact that a visual idea may be the same idea as an organic idea. It may be even doubted that such a thing as an organic idea exists. But we may suppose, for the sake of argument, that every visual idea has its organic correspondent, which is quite similar to the concept expressed above, in other words, that every visual idea has its motor form. We might just as well say that every visual idea had its auditory form, and every olfactory idea had its auditory form and so on, throughout the entire list of twenty odd qualities of sensation.

How does the visual idea get its motor form? How does it get its organic form? What does it mean when we say that a visual idea has a motor form? It cannot mean anything else than that the visual idea, or visual impression, is inherently and by heredity associated with the motion. That this is the case can hardly be doubted. Imitation of action is necessary for collective action in herds, flights, swarms, shoals, droves and other social units, that act as a unit without thinking individually. The fish in a shoal all swimming rapidly in one direction, and turning in unison, if obstructed or frightened, are manifestly guided by visual impressions. The visual impression instantly issues in appropriate action. The action is the motor form of the visual impression or visual idea.

The infant in the cradle will smile if it sees a smile, and wave its arms in imitation of arms or other moving things. Before three years of age the elaborate mechanism of speech, largely imitative, is the motor form of an auditory impression. It is one of the many miracles of human activity. That a child should instinctively use a set of muscles in lips, throat and lungs (muscles which it can neither see nor separately feel), successfully to reproduce a sound which it has heard, is no more surprising, when "curiously considered" than that any impression of any sense quality should have any form whatever in any other sense quality.

Now in the emotions we have an instinctive motor reaction, a behaviour pattern, which is determined partly by external and partly by internal impressions. An emotion is the motor or organic form of a visual, an auditory or any other sense quality of idea. This is very clear in the case of the emotions we call love. The organic or motor form of the visual idea, and particularly of the tactual, cutaneous, olfactory and thermal ideas, is a reflex of the sense idea of vision, just as is the baby's imitative act in smiling the motor form of the visual idea. And it is the same idea, only in another form.

The point chiefly to be emphasized in all this is that the motor reaction or organic reaction is more frequently than not an entirely unconscious matter. Only when the reactions have been accumulated in summation to a degree which shakes the whole body do we speak of them as conscious emotions. Only at a certain intensity do they burst into consciousness and draw our attention to them alone. And then they completely upset us, and we do not know how to handle them. We are as if unconscious ourselves of all else save the emotion, and the so-called "expression" of it is generally so far outside of our conscious control that we "are not ourselves." Contemporary psychologists define the emotions as reflexes that "interrupt" the ordinary stream of consciousness, and reserve the term emotion for the interruption, maintaining that there is no such thing as an unconscious emotion.

But the emotions of love are the organic and

motor reactions to the total situation, a situation chiefly constituted by the presence (remembered or imagined) of a member of the other sex. Furthermore, like most of our mental life, they are more unconscious than conscious. That is, they carry on their activities in consciousness less frequently than in various depths of the unconscious.

It will appear, too, as we proceed, that not only is love not one emotion but many emotions, but also it is, in all of its passionate forms, more active in the unconscious than it is in consciousness. Thus we shall have to speak of conscious passion, but quite as much of unconscious passion, the latter being quite as real and quite as active as the former, and infinitely more extensive, involving as it does practically every atom of tissue in the human body.

" Love " may be an auditory word, a visual word, a motor word; it may be an auditory idea, a visual idea, a motor idea. In the human mind-body incorporation love is however only sometimes a word but more frequently it takes other forms, now an organic impression, now a muscular activity. So protean is it that it may and does take any form of impression or expression (sensation or action) of which the human psychophysical incorporation is capable. In a happy child it takes the form of ebullition of spirits showing itself in almost every act and word and tone of voice, even in the little rages in which, however, it is transmuted instantaneously into hate. In the child it is body-wide and yet not unified.

In the adult who has had forced on him by society some, at least, of his multifarious activities, love may be very much disguised. It may be transmuted into fear, anger, hate, and, paradoxically enough, into disease, which is a form of fear. If the outward motor expressive form of love be well developed in infancy or early childhood, it is not so likely to be transformed later into hate, fear or other disease, for habit rules in this as in other forms of behaviour. Love is that organic motor form of the libido which finds its expression in deeds that harmonize most with the progress of development of the social unit, be that as large as it may. Love, therefore, transformed into a phobia, is an irrational and an archaic form, transformed into crime or madness, still more archaic. Transformed into its highest form, it inspires the individual to deeds that connect him with each member of wider and wider circles of social co-operation. Its being limitless enables it to be drawn upon to warm the heart and fire the imagination to include every one in the world, and it rouses the individual to activities which seem to others heroic in magnitude.

It is, however, only potentially limitless, for, in actual life, it stops with husband or wife, brother or sister, father or mother, neighbour or fellow citizen as the case may be, the line being drawn wherever the individual becomes unable to *feel* properly toward the person in question.

In the individual psychophysical incorporation it should extend to and animate every atom of tissue, and it should be so lively as to enter consciousness spontaneously in every minute of waking life and in the dream life of sleep. It should enter consciousness in its own true form, which is that of acceptive, integrative power, the power to create cosmic unities, where before existed only chaotic multiplicities. But in humans individually it is transformed into far other forms that externally do not in the least resemble it. A phobia is a much disguised form of love. A headache is a sadly transmuted form of love, for it is generally a form of self-love, which is caused by the object being changed from external to internal.

In the case of a phobia, the love is so disguised as to be absolutely unrecognizable. It may therefore be properly called unconscious. As love, it does not enter consciousness. All the individual is conscious of is a fear of knives, snakes, lightning, tunnels, closed places, open places, etc. Every one of those fears, however, is a transmuted desire to create. In the unconscious it is a desire, in conscious life it is a fear. The fear is conscious; the desire is unconscious. The fear is a transmutation of the desire, and only the transmutation appears to view.

In compulsions it is transformed into acts which enter consciousness together with a feeling that it is not only compulsive but inexplicable or even irrational. Compulsive doubt is a conscious form of an absolutely unconscious trend of the libido.

D. *Pleasure-Pain vs. Reality*

Two principles govern human activity, that called the pleasure-pain principle, and that called the reality principle. According to the first we instinctively accept the pleasurable and reject the painful. According to the second we accept some painful experiences, because in so doing we follow an ideal which is imposed upon us from without by society or by the world of things. The second is as much the result of living in physical relations with other people and things, as the first is innate and spontaneous.

The desires arising out of the unconscious craving, and given definite shape by external experiences, are frustrated repeatedly by other persons and things, by the fact that other persons would be pained or angered by our gratification of our unconscious craving, and that real things stand in our way. Thus comes the connection between pain and the unconscious, shown in the fact that the unconscious is not only the origin of impulses whose carrying out would be painful, but is also the repository or scrap heap for conscious experiences that have proved painful, unpleasant or disappointing.

The result of this has been to give a sort of black eye to the unconscious, and make some people regard it as something to be carefully let alone—shunned as a graveyard of dead hopes and defunct wishes. Of course, in a sense, it *is* our enemy, or the antagonist of a conscious part of ourselves, but the best fight against any opponent is made by those who know the opponent thoroughly. The results of regarding the unconscious as something to be shunned are most disastrous, producing, as this attitude does, many human ills, both physical and mental. A further result of it is the fact that the desires bred of the unconscious craving upon the things of the external world are, by virtue of the forces of consciousness and the foreconscious, kept repressed in their original, crass, literal form, and are only allowed to enter consciousness in the form of some visual, auditory or other idea acceptable to society. The other ideas, acceptable to society, are, for an unnecessarily large number of people, neuroses, diseases, eccentricities, mental disorders. The neuroses, diseases, etc., are the physiological forms of the organic and motor ideas, which are in turn forms of still other (visual, auditory, etc.,) ideas. What drives an idea from one form into another, is the unconscious life force, which has been given the name of libido, and the obstructions which that life force meets, now here, now there, in its centrifugal path of expression. Denied one outlet, it naturally, like rising water, seeks another. Thus we can say that the auditory idea is another form of a visual idea or of a motor idea, and so on, because they are all merely expressions of the one libido force—the vital energy ever turning latent into free energy. Blocked in one avenue toward action, it takes the next higher egress toward the external world, and as impartially and inevitably as the tide rising in an estuary.

Taking the next higher egress implies that like water, the libido never rises beyond its lowest outlet. In order to get it to rise, the lower ones have to be stopped. Sources of satisfaction are graded by society as high or low. The work of education is centred about the stopping of the lower ones, and opening of higher outlets for the libido. Autoerotism is the lowest outlet, if it can be called an outlet, as the object of the desires of the libido in autoerotic gratification is the individual himself, body or soul. The highest outlet is that affecting most of the world of external reality—persons and things. The activities of mind and body thus directed upon externals are true reality thinking, and always aim to change something in external reality.

The unconscious mental activities are, therefore, so associated with pain or displeasure, which is indeed sometimes the contribution to them of the very fact of the individual's living in a social organization, that they do not enter consciousness except in disguise. This is of the nature of a symbolism.* The unconscious activities themselves do not enter, but symbols representing them do. Here we come again upon the matter of the manifestations of unconscious passion. Such manifestations are generally but symbols of the passion itself, as it does not manifest itself literally, except in the most intimate relations of men and women.

E. *The Total Situation Contains Unconscious Passion.*

So eating love
Inhabits in the finest wits of all.
Two Gentlemen of Verona, I, 1, 43.

When a man or a woman is in love, a part of their total mental and physical situation is not

* See Wilfrid Lay, *Man's Unconscious Conflict,* page 67.

consciously perceptible. In the ardour of conscious passion undoubtedly more mental activities than usual emerge into consciousness, and people are more alive in the sense of being aware of what is going on in their minds than when they are not thus ardent. Even so, there is a large amount of mental activity of which they are not, and cannot become, conscious.

In people, on the other hand, who are not consciously in love, there is, either repressed or not directly manifest, an unconscious passion. It is the most powerful factor in all human activity, and everybody is practically violently in love all the time with some other person or imaginary personality, even though their actually visible deportment shows to the uninitiated nothing of this. We are all in love constantly, whether we know it or not. We show it clearly to the initiated. If we are not aware that we are in love, we are still in love,—and with a definite person. Who is it, and how can we find out who it is? * Can we, after finding out, make love to her or him, and make them reciprocate? Do we unconsciously know this so well that we consciously hide the fact from ourselves, lest we be consciously disappointed? We should be honest

* It will later be shown that in many cases the woman with whom the man is in love, is his own mother as she appeared to him when he was less than five years of age.

enough to admit this, and to believe that unconscious disappointment is more serious for us than conscious disappointment.

If a man was shown that he was in love with a certain woman, and replied that it was better for him not to know it consciously, because she was happily married, what should we tell him then? We could tell him that there is still some other woman to whom he can direct his conscious passion, and that if the unconscious passion was not soon thereafter transferred to her, it would be because his unconscious passion was attached not to a real person, but to an idea. This is quite contrary to the notion that marriages are made in heaven, and that for every man there is just one woman in the world that can make him supremely happy. But this truth is best expressed conversely, that supreme happiness can be obtained by a man only through complete devotion to one woman, as long as she lives a woman, or by a woman only through complete devotion to one man.

Described in modern psychological terms, the unconscious passion, which exists in every individual, can, by the proper methods, be completely and permanently transferred to any one of a comparatively large number of eligible mates; but the single devotion to the single individual is the only perfect type of love, which is the only one that completely fills and satisfies the life.

The notion that only one woman in the world can completely satisfy the life instinct of any given man and vice versa is thus seen to be a slightly perverted form of the notion that a man should attach himself only to one woman. The latter is true, the former is false,—as false as that only one special copy of a book would be pleasant to read, all the others of the same printing being unpleasant to read.

As has been suggested above, the total situation that gives the man the notion that only a certain individual woman can fill his life, and that no other can, is one in which there is a crystallization into an unchangeable idea, a condition that indicates lifelessness and not life in the man.

It will be shown in the following pages that in many people this crystallization has abnormally taken place at a very early age, and that such people go about looking for the real person who will match this fixed photographic negative that is in their own souls, and sometimes unsuccessfully try many experiments, little knowing that the fixed negative is the imprint on their souls of their father or mother, or some other relative, and that normal humans should have no such fixed negative. True mating implies a conscious and an unconscious adaptation, which in turn requires that each one of a pair should have enough elasticity and adaptability to mate with the other fully. Yet frequently two people marry, each with a fixed negative that does not at all match the other person.

F. *Reciprocal Impressions*

When a man and a woman are conversing, impressions are being made constantly upon the unconscious of the man, both by the conscious acts and words of the woman and by her unconscious acts. Also the consciousness of the man may perceive both what the woman consciously does and says, and what she unconsciously does and says.

Conversely impressions are constantly made upon the unconscious of the woman by the conscious acts and words of the man and by his unconscious acts and words. Also the conscious mind of the woman may perceive not only what the man consciously says and does, but also what he unconsciously says and does.

We might illustrate this with a man and a woman sitting in separate boats ten feet apart on clear water ten feet deep. Below the man is an eel; below the woman is a fish. Now (1) the man can clearly see the woman, can dimly see the

eel below him and can less easily see the fish
under the woman's boat. (2) The woman can
clearly see the man, next the fish and least clearly
the eel. (3) But the eel can see the boat the
man is in, can see the boat the woman is in and
can also see the fish. (4) Similarly the fish
can clearly see the eel, less clearly the boat the
woman is in, and least clearly the boat the man
is in.

Expressing this another way, the eel is impressed by sensations coming from the man, the
woman and the fish, the fish is impressed by sensations coming from the eel, the man and the
woman. Likewise the man has three sources of
impression, and so does the woman. But the
unconscious of the man is represented by the
eel, that of the woman by the fish. In other
words, the eel is a part of the man and the
fish is a part of the woman, in our illustration. The eel in every man, so to speak, can
see not only what the man is doing but also what
the woman is doing, who in this illustration
represents the conscious life of the woman, and
what the fish, representing the unconscious life
of the woman, is doing. Furthermore the eel of
the man can perceive through all the senses
of the man what the fish of the woman is doing.

Expressing this in another way and amplifying it, the man reacts to the eel, the woman and

the fish; the eel reacts to the man, the woman and
the fish; the woman reacts to the eel, the man
and the fish; and the fish to the man, the woman
and the eel. Literally the conscious mind of the
man reacts to the conscious mind of the woman,
to the unconscious mind (eel) of the man and to
the unconscious mind (fish) of the woman. The
conscious mind of the woman reacts to the other
three factors, and so do the unconscious minds
of the man and the woman react to the corresponding three other factors in the present situation. And they are all doing it all the time, not
only in each other's presence, but *in absentia;*
the conscious and the unconscious mind and
body of each are reacting to the conscious and
unconscious impressions previously made by the
mind and body of the other.

And as the conscious mind of each of them is
made up of impressions and thoughts streaming
in from all of the twenty odd different sources of
sensation, eyes, ears, noses, skin, muscles, internal organs, etc., so is the unconscious mind of
each of them made up of impressions constantly
received from each and every one of the same
sources of sensation, in every way, exactly like
the conscious impressions, except that neither
man nor woman is conscious of them.

What the man consciously says or does is perfectly patent to the man. What he unconsciously

says, he may never know at all, as when he talks in his sleep, when he says things in a rage and sometimes when he makes an ordinary slip of the tongue. For example, a man was telling me how deeply affected a woman was by a play to which he had taken her, saying that she even cried all the way home in the subway train. As I did not mention his error, he probably does not yet know that he called it the " sob "-way train. In short, very few, if any, of us know at the time all that we are actually doing, though our senses are reporting it constantly to our minds, and some of us do not know all we have said. We all act and speak unconsciously all the time; so do we think unconsciously all the time.

Similarly feeling goes on in us all the time, whether we are conscious of it or not.

In illustrating the foregoing, I might have said that the foot of the man perceives what the foot of the woman is doing quite as well as that the eye of the man sees what the eye of the woman is doing and conversely. But then I should have had to tell how a foot can perceive, which is not thought of as a perceiving organ, except by touch, which is ruled out because they are ten feet apart.

But it has been lately shown that tensions in muscles of the foot (and in every other muscle) may be set up by the visual perception of what another's foot may be doing at the time.

It is pointed out that these muscular contractions, and continued states of muscular contraction, technically called the " postural tonus," are equivalent to unconscious mental activities, so that properly to " understand " a ballet, for example, one has to have parallel contractions in one's own body corresponding to the movements of the dancer one is looking at.

This will explain the great allurement of the baseball or football game. The hundreds of thousands of spectators are not only literally making movements that reproduce in little the movements of the players, and thus are identifying themselves in the most intimate way with the winners, but they are also literally carrying out motions that the players themselves have not the time to carry out,—motions, I mean, that are the expression of the emotions. The same is true in the audiences of all the moving picture shows night and day all over the country. They sit apparently still, but with their bodies acutely a-quiver as they minutely reproduce in themselves the movements of the actors on the screen. The same is true of all spectators of every spectacular performance, of every parade, play or what not, that focuses the attention of large numbers of people. The lack of success of a play is due to the inability of the actors, whether from lack of good acting of from faulty dramatic construction, to "put across" the footlights just these imitative motions, drunk in by the eyes of the audience and, without the audience's consciously knowing it, reproduced in their sympathetic contractions of their bodies in unison with those of the actors'.*

These involuntary movements occasionally become magnified enough to be perceptible to others. The becoming conscious of them is sometimes a source of much amusement or of painful embarrassment. When shaking hands some people give involuntary expression to their unconscious desires by a slight push away from, or a pull toward, themselves of the other person's hand, a push or pull of which they are not themselves aware. The other person frequently observes this, though he (or she) may not understand it. Certain "breaks" in ordinary conversation show the same involuntary expression of the unconscious desire. For instance, Ruggles asks Gerry who is the author of certain stories now being circulated about Ruggles. Gerry may reply: "I don't know, really, Paterson, who it is," naming the very person whom he wished to shield, and showing how strong was the unconscious desire on Gerry's part to tell Ruggles, stronger indeed than his conscious wish to keep the secret.

* See Kempf, *The Autonomic Functions and the Personality*, 1918.

Unconscious passion is exactly this thing, only carried out along erotic lines. The eye of the youth, beholding the alluring beauty of the maiden as she walks and moves, instinctively arouses, by virtue of accumulated associations, inherited through thousands of years of evolution, a system of infinitesimal muscular contractions, in both involuntary and voluntary muscles. These sometimes never enter his consciousness, or if they do, they enter as an indescribable yearning to fondle her, or as a series of actions unaccountable to himself and to her. This behaviour of his and how she consciously reacts to it is all that is manifest to either of them at the time, but it is of far less importance for their future welfare than that of which they are unconscious. And this is the case whether they ever go any farther than merely looking at each other, and saying a few inconsiderable things.

For it is the unconscious reaction on his part and hers that determines whether they are to be happy or tragically wretched if ever they marry. The sum total of all these organic reactions, movements or tonuses in the muscles of the arms, legs, trunk, etc., and in the involuntary muscles of heart, lungs, blood and other vessels and glands, is the physical substratum, if it is not itself literally, the unconscious passion which we have been considering.

The unconscious passion is thus seen to be a sort of muscular " set " of both kinds of muscles, determined by a disposition of cells in the brain and nerves, and indirectly on verbal and other ideas which integrate them.   E.g. when Juliet says: " Wherefore art thou Romeo? " and that a rose by any other name would smell as sweet, she is expressing only an unconscious wish that it would, knowing full well that it does not; and the state of society in which the two lovers grew up was the cause of their tragic end, just on account of the power of the two words Capulet and Montague to enlist so much of their activities, and thus form so much of their fate.

Helena: Love looks not with the eyes but with the mind;
And therefore is wing'd Cupid painted blind:
Nor hath Love's mind of any judgment taste;
Wings and no eyes figure unheedy haste:
And therefore is Love said to be a child,
Because in choice he is so oft beguil'd.
Midsummer Night's Dream, I, 1, 234.

CHAPTER II

A. *Civilization and Passion*

UNCONSCIOUS passion is the crassly sexual concupiscence that has caused so much prudery as an over-compensation in civilized peoples, who have, as a rule, not understood the difference between repressing it and controlling it. Ancient Greek thought represented it as something necessary only for procreation, and regarded the average woman as a child-bearing mechanism merely. Sex was therefore debased by them in comparison with the transfer of the conscious passion to something other than woman, the natural object of it. With the Greek man the object of the conscious passion was another man, but it is not to be supposed that his unconscious passion was any more than merely hoodwinked by the homosexual practices. Roman civilization generally placed the woman on a higher level than the Greek, at the same time putting no limitations practically on promiscuity, except for legal status of families. In the fall of the Roman civilization and through the Middle Ages, pagan brutality in sex ran parallel with Christian asceticism. In the type of society in which flourished the Courts of Love the crassly sexual passion was frankly indulged in with one class of women, while another class was set upon a pedestal and to it was attributed the ascetic purity which had been the ideal of some leaders of Christian morality.

In all this there was a duality and a contrast emphasized between heavenly and earthly love,— a contrast which is apparent today in the attitude of civilization toward the crassly sexual. Each individual recognizes two natures struggling within himself, but society, in attempting to control the so-called lower, instinctive nature, has used the only method with which it was acquainted—repression. This is due to the essential infantility of society's attitude toward the race-perpetuating instinct. It is only very recently that methods of birth control have been generally known and tentatively practised, methods which will enable man to control the instinct itself and to employ for his own ennoblement the most powerful force in Nature. Civilization up to date has not ennobled mankind, for no calm observer, noting the events of the past decade, can regard mankind as in general anything but extremely ignoble. There will be no real progress made until man avails himself socially of all his enormous reproductive power, and ceases to waste it in disorders, social, mental and physical, which are the indirect manifestations of the repressed sexual desires.

The fact that society has only raised obstruction against and not taken control of the manifestation of natural instincts (and only certain instincts at that), is proof of society's ineptness and puerility in going at the thing from the wrong end. To stop a leak, society roughly plasters a patch on the outside of a reservoir, plugs a hole in a dam from the outside, instead of from the inside, where the pressure of the water would help to hold the plug in place. This externality and superficiality of all society's efforts to conserve human power is in sharp contrast to the scientific methods, which have produced such remarkable results in material progress in modern times. Whatever force and intelligence have been applied by mankind to the production of machinery and chemical agencies have been applied only there, and have as yet been very slightly used in the development of the forces of life itself.

In the individual human life a fountain of power is constantly upspringing, which society has only blindly organized,—has, indeed, with a sort of nonagenarian anile fluster, merely tried to gloze over on the outside. All legislation is of a flatly and supinely repressive character, a culmination of which is seen in the prohibition of drugs, alcohol, etc. While the fable of the sun and the wind is an ancient one, its application to social life has been most sporadic, and, where applied, the sun has been so enveloped in wind that the resistance of mankind has been developed and his development retarded. For example, the Y.M.C.A. and Y.W.C.A. and all other such bodies are a groping in the direction of developing the character by drawing out, as with sunshine, the powers of man, as the leaves are drawn out of the buds by the sunlight of a warm May day. But with this eliciting there goes so much negation in the matter of what the young men and women must *not* do, as almost entirely to vitiate the possible unspeakably good results. In the recreation movement there is much good being done in enlisting the powers of men and women in creative social work, but the effects of this work will not be manifest to all persons until the entire population takes up the movement and insists on public funds being devoted to creating attractive and desirable conditions, outside of actual working conditions, also, in all localities of the country.

The two natures, struggling within the individual, can be, and must be, reconciled, so that the individual may become the unity he has never yet been except in the rarest of isolated cases.

The reproductive instinct is absolutely natural, normal, wholesome and if properly controlled, ennobling; and alone able to develop man and woman into finer members of society than have yet been produced.

Unconscious passion is at least partly the work of repression effected by civilization in its infantile attempts to control by means of annihilation. But it is quite evident that annihilation is the opposite of control. Society that sees the annihilation of the sexual instinct as the only means of reshaping it is exactly in the position of the infant which shuts its eyes to a blinding light because it cannot turn it down, or throws away anything because it cannot reshape that thing or use it. If society had been successful in this attempt to annihilate, civilized peoples would have annihilated themselves.

Therefore fear has been the emotion dominant in society. Fear is dispelled by knowledge, and knowledge about the psychology of the sexual instinct is being rapidly collected by science and today for the first time is being disseminated not only through private but through national channels, witness the activities of the U. S. Bureaus of Education and Public Health.

As society has repressed the direct manifestations of the reproductive instinct, the individual has been deprived of a direct consciousness of them and their direct effect, which is much more wholesome than their indirect result, has had a veil drawn over it, so that the work of centuries has now to be done over again.

The repression of the sexual instinct begins at a very early age in the individual and results not only in indirect manifestations of the instinct taking the place of direct ones, but also in the indirect manifestations not being recognized for what they really are, and in the various forms of perverted vision and perception generally, and in individual instances of mental disorder so great as to result in serious economic waste.

The worst result of the repression of the sexual instinct into the unconscious of man, and particularly of woman, is that it effectively undermines the wholesomeness of family life, on which is based both individual happiness and the prosperity of the race. I shall show very clearly that the repression of this instinct in one or both parties to a marriage is the cause of prostitution, of divorce and of most of the ills from which society now suffers.

For nowadays a couple generally marry absolutely without proper knowledge of the physiology and particularly of the psychology of the sexual emotions. Usually neither of them knows whether their unconscious passion is directed toward each other, and sometimes for so-called economic reasons they marry with neither affection nor conscious passion. I shall attempt to show in the following pages that the marriages in which either or both are lacking are productive of misery that might have been avoided.

Thus there are many total situations in family life that are quite destructive of the individual's possibility of making so successful a marital union that both conscious and unconscious passion can be permanently transferred. As such total situations I might first mention the families in which there is but one child. There is here a double misfortune, for not only does the mother love the child too much, but the child loves the mother too much. As will be later explained, love is made up of affection and passion, and while affection in the strict sense cannot generally be overdone, passion can, and, in the single-child family is usually over-stressed. The only thing that can save many such children from an early crystallization in which their love takes on a " fixed negative " form, is to send them away to school or to adopt other children, who will help withstand the lightning blast of too concentrated parental love. Much of this love takes the form of unconscious passion and therefore passes beyond control of either parent or child, forming the fixed photographic negative that causes the future unhappiness of the child by rendering impossible his or her necessary adaptation to a future spouse.

B. *A Woman's Unconscious Passion*

Most men's unconscious passion, being generally either sublimated or directly gratified, is less evident in their ordinary actions than is woman's. Any kind of kittenishness in women (in public) is a manifestation of unconscious passion. In private, that is, with their husbands or lovers, they can be as playful as possible, and their playfulness will only be an added charm to their manners. But a woman is kittenish just as she is cattish, from unconscious reasons. She is kittenish, with a person not husband or lover, either because literally she has neither husband or lover, or because figuratively she does not possess them fully. If she had complete happiness in her husband or lover, she would reserve for him all her playfulness, because, being fully transferred to him, she can feel in his company alone that these preliminaries to an embrace are appropriate. If she cannot be playful with her husband, because for example he has a frown " set " in the concrete of his ossified soul, she lacks just that amount of emotional outlet in the very place where it ought to be let out, and, in order to get the satisfaction of the portion of her unconscious passion that has been admitted to these paths of expression she must be playful in the company of some other man than the stern and dignified husband.

Therefore, if she is young, and her husband middle aged, she will surround herself with young college men, with whom she will carry on all sorts of flirtations. If she is rich, she will take them on long afternoon and evening rides in her car, she will entertain them in her home in the country, and in private rooms in hotels in the city, loading them with presents, and being hugely gratified by their animal spirits, all of which arouse her unconscious passion, but quite without her knowing it, or being willing to admit the fact. Her husband, who does his part in the family with decorum and unimpeachable good humour, is not in the least jealous of her, consciously at any rate, nor does she violate sexual morality in any way, her most flagrant offence having been that she opened the door of her room in the hotel and kissed one of her young admirers good-bye one morning after he had spent the night in another room as her guest. In the hurry of parting she partially forgot that she was dressed only in her *robe de nuit!*

Her actions' effect on her young college men friends is another matter entirely. What impressions may be made by her behaviour on the unconscious mental reactions of the boys themselves is easily to be surmised. To be taken into the home of an attractive woman, only a dozen or so years older than they, to be dined and wined by her at expensive hotels in the city, can not fail to be a strong factor in arousing their unconscious passion. They are in one sense quite as ignorant as she of the results caused in the largest areas of their personalities. They may know they desire her person, but her irreproachable conduct when they have been so bold as to attempt to go too far with her, has been as a steel wall to their farther advances. In this she is playing adorable mother to them, and is putting exactly the same barrier between herself and them as do their own mothers. No wonder their mothers are extremely jealous of this erratic woman, who, having only two children and ample means for a dozen of her own, is compensating for her small family of own children by enlarging her number of foster children. That they are all boys is a direct proof of the fact that it is her unconscious sexual passion that she is gratifying in this harmless (?) vicarious manner.

Under the guise of affection, which society approves, this woman is carrying on at a great rate with young men for whom she would not naturally feel affection, but biologically should feel passion, if she allowed them to come so close to her. And they, being in the vigorously experimental epoch of their development, rely solely upon her to prevent them from going too far with her. They too are acting under the guise of affection, but dominated by their own unconscious passion.

I give this illustration here because it is one of those episodes that would ordinarily be attributed by the woman herself to mere affection, though the total situation is one ordinarily of unconscious passion on both sides, under particularly aggravating circumstances, which are saved from actual immorality only by the vigorous repression on the part of the woman herself.

C. *Conscious Passion*

> My love doth so approve him
> That even his stubbornness, his checks, and frowns
> Have grace and favour in them.
> *Othello*, IV, 3, 20.

Conscious passion is not difficult to recognize or to describe. It is that portion of the emotions connected with the love instinct of which the man or woman is fully aware. Running alongside of and behind it is, however, in some cases an indefinite feeling that all is, or is not, harmonious. For the youth or maiden whose unconscious passion is directed to the other, the other should be absolutely perfect. Even her caprices should be wholly approved. Even his roughness and lack of tact should be completely acceptable. The grace and favour of the checks and frowns are the contribution of the unconscious passion. In those persons, however, whose conscious passion is not founded upon the unconscious passion there will be little incidents in their mutual life, particularly if they regard each other as possible mates,—incidents that seem puzzlingly inconsistent with the expression, as they see it, of the conscious passion of each for the other. These are traits apparently trivial, such as slight mannerisms, habits, forgetfulness, dislikes or mild aversions, which singly are as drops of water, or straws in the wind showing a direction in the unconscious passion at variance with the clearly perceived conscious passion.

The fact that these trivial circumstances enter the consciousness of either of the two is the external manifestation of an unconscious doubt. No couple should marry if there is the slightest reservation expressed or implied on either side.

The implied reservations are the feelings unconsciously aroused in the woman, which make some of the inconsequential acts of the man take on so much importance as to be consciously noticed at all, and the feelings of which the man is quite unconscious, but which cause him to become *unpleasantly* aware of some slight imperfection in the woman.

Finally it should be understood that absolutely everything that is not an expression of conscious passion between them *is* an expression of the *unconscious* passion that they may be having for some other person or imaginary personality. If all is well, no act of either is in any way unacceptable to the other. If any act of either does produce an unpleasant reaction in the other, all is not well. In such a case, the unconscious passion of one of them is not wholly directed to the other. The reaction then may be the most indefinite feeling of unrest unassociated with any concrete idea. But no matter how indefinite it is, it is enough. They should not marry, until there is no such feeling.

Sometimes the unrest comes from a real or fancied disapproval of their choice, on the part of parents or relatives. If, however, unrest from this source is very great, it argues that the unconscious passion is too firmly fixed upon the family, either when it is a real disapproval, because love that scorns walls of stone should not be brooked with family ties, or when it is a fancied one, the disapproval is still the unconscious bond that inhibits the individual from forming close ties outside of the family. Many marriages should be delayed until the betrothed have lived a sufficiently long time apart from their families, for such family ties to become disintegrated, without which disintegration, no perfect union can take place, involving as it should the complete transfer of both conscious and unconscious passion.

The indefinite feelings are some of the outward signs of unconscious passion. The more indefinite, the more surely are they the signs of unconscious, and not of conscious, passion. The only way to make them definite, and therefore to make them conscious, is to think about them. To sit in meditation for at least thirty minutes a day, and to admit freely to consciousness whatever thoughts *suggest themselves,* exercising no selection and resolutely refusing to fear, or to be repelled by, any of them. Whatever they may be, they represent, even though symbolically, the individual as he or she, in the largest areas of personality, really is. Thus it appears that even conscious passion may contain, in the indefinite feelings experienced at the time, the elements of unconscious passion. The unconscious passion is the background showing through, the background of uneasiness and unrest, where the unconscious is at variance with the conscious, but, where they are harmonious, the unconscious passion is the source of the golden light that suffuses all of love's experiences.

We shall have to look at unconscious passion from several angles, and in one of these it is necessary to make a distinction between affection, which is never unconscious, and passion, which in the most highly civilized persons, is more unconscious than conscious.

CHAPTER III

A. *The Stream of Life*

OF the stream of life, there are two component currents, affection and passion. Affection comes from the emotions of the earliest dawn of life within the womb and is directed primarily toward the mother, from whom the child receives not only life and its sole support for months, but also, after that, receives the greater part of its joys, its comforts, and its pleasures of every kind. In infancy, the other current, passion, is a dew upon the uplands of individual life, which is absorbed by the sun of childhood's days and descends in a mighty shower upon the adolescent at the time when down appears upon the upper lip of the boy and the breasts of the girl round out to the lines of greatest beauty.

Soon the boy becomes a man, but even before this his passion has been instinctively directed toward his mother. Being naturally without insight, and knowing nothing intuitively about the impropriety of feeling passion toward his mother, he gives expression to this naïvely. He does some little thing showing an unconscious passion for his mother, who, having some insight, recognizes it at once and rejects it. He sees her, for example, in her undergarments and presses his cheek against her breast, or he puts her bare arms around his neck, or he says how beautiful she is. Whereupon the mother feels an impulse born of her own unconscious passion for him and of the knowledge that passion of son for mother is not right. She tells him not to give expression to those thoughts about her. If he asks her toward whom then he should feel passion, she tells him for no one at present, but that he should wait until he is married as those feelings are only for a husband to express to his wife. She thereby represses in him the passion which, if she is completely successful, will never be expressed in the right way again.

For it is a recently discovered psychological law that the object toward which an original passion is directed, can never be replaced if the desire be not gratified, but be unconditionally repressed. Therefore, there is every reason why a mother should not be allowed to become the original object of passion for the boy, or the father for the girl. It would be much better if the child were taken away from its own parents at a very early age, and placed in an environment where the first object of passion could not be a person against whom society has reared the incest barrier. For the inhibitions thus formed will adhere to all the persons otherwise eligible for a love mate. Passion being turned back from the mother, toward whom in some men it happens by force of circumstances to be directed, will ever afterward, because of this very fact, be turned away unconsciously from all women that have the mother's social stamp, for example, sisters, cousins, sisters' friends, and any girl who could be regarded as a mother's, or sister's equal or surrogate.

If the mother's warning to the son that he should not entertain those feelings toward her or toward his sister is worded in such a way as to give the erroneous impression, that passion itself should be felt for no women, it will be understood to apply, frequently, only to women of the mother's class and not to women who have a shady character. It thus results that the boy's passion is not repressed entirely, for it is almost impossible definitively to repress so strong a current of feeling, but it is diverted from women of the mother-sister class to the demi-monde. This applies to passion and not to affection.

Affection, on the other hand, is not touched by the incest barrier. It is cultivated by society as an oil which lubricates. Affection may be felt for mother and sister, for father and brother, for

house and home, and horse and dog, for food
and drink, amusements and recreations and all
the physical means of carrying them out.

A distinction of great importance between affection and passion is that passion may be both
conscious and unconscious, while affection is
never anything but conscious. Therefore, in the
combinations of passion, with and without insight * on the part of men and women or both
we shall not have to consider affection at all.
It is only unconscious passion that, with imperceptible bonds, binds the man to a self-made
ideal of his own mother, and unconscious passion
that binds the woman by the same imperceptible
bonds to the ideal she has herself made though
unconsciously, of her father's personality.

B. *The Parent Imago*

This ideal is known as the parent imago,
(mother imago or father imago, as the case may
be), but they both contain passion, not affection.
Affection is more nearly connected with the instinct for self-preservation; passion is the expression of the race-preservative instinct. Affection is the feeling of gratitude or comfort coming
from the receipt of nourishment at the mother's
breast; it is the feelings of gratification experi-

* See chapter IV.

enced by the child when it is lifted, held in lap, hugged, washed, put to bed, allowed to creep into parents' bed, when it is given any food or drink or amusement and when it is given any satisfaction of its needs of growth of body or mind.   It is naturally most felt toward those who do most for the child, but it is felt also toward all other persons who please the child in any way.   And it is always conscious.   It always implies the receipt of a favour, and is a feeling which in some natures will be worked out into external expression naturally in a favour returned.   But there is in it no thought of giving spontaneously, or of complete sacrifice, a feeling which is characteristic only of passion.   This is one of the reasons why the expression of affection is so consciously cultivated by men and women, and why it may be wholesomely felt by man for man and by woman for woman.   But passion is never wholesomely felt by men for men or by women for women.

People in short always know when they feel affection for other persons or things, but they frequently do not know when they feel passion for other persons.   Furthermore, it will appear in what follows, that conscious passion for one person may go along with unconscious passion for quite a different person, or for no person really existing, but for an ideal or imago of a

mother or father. This mother imago which attracts to itself the unconscious passion of the
son is something that exists solely in the unconscious mind of the son himself, and is associated
by contiguity with the mother, but only as she
existed from ten to forty or even fifty years ago;
with the result that the love life of some men is
dominated by a group of impressions made long
ago and which the present woman named mother,
could not possibly produce. Many times therefore, a man is unconsciously in love, that is, his
unconscious passion is directed toward, the imago
of a woman who is dead—an unconscious mem-
ory of one who no longer lives.

That this imago (a Latin word for ghost)
should make it impossible for a man to have
children, is to be sure a gruesome thought, but
it is in some cases literally true, and at other
times true of legitimate, while not of illegitimate,
children; where for instance, the mother imago
prevents the married man from having children
from his wife, but not from a prostitute, or other
woman of shady character, not in his wife's
social position.

An unconscious passion for the mother, on the
man's part, or for the father on the woman's
part, called the Œdipus * or Electra complex
respectively, is a much commoner fact than one
    * See § H of this chapter.

would believe possible, and it is the reason for many degrees of marital unhappiness ranging all the way from gradually increasing indifference on the part of one or the other of the pair, to all-embracing hatred or impotence on the part of one or both of them.

It is as if the unconscious passion toward the parent imago lay above and weighed down the unconscious passion for any other man or woman that might later be met. Or it is as if the unconscious passion for the mother imago got in the way of the man's vision of any other woman, so that, as it were, he can see any woman with whom he may later become acquainted, only through a screen made up of his memories of, and phantasies about, his mother. This prevents him for seeing the wife *as she really is,* for it will be evident that, as the mother originally disclaimed any sexual feelings, the boy, and later the same man, sees all women through this mother imago screen with the red rays of sexual passion filtered out of them.

C. *Effect of the Imago Screen*

All impressions received through such a screen are intensified if they are like, or are imperceptible if they are unlike, the picture made by the shape of the screen. Therefore to a man with a vivid unconscious mother imago, all girls unlike the mother fail to make an impression of such a kind as to arouse the unconscious passion; but girls who are like the mother, do arouse this unconscious passion in so far as they resemble this unconscious imago. The passion of the man here described, is directed solely to this unconscious imago of his mother, and is finally and permanently fixated there, so that if a woman is partially identified with it through greater or less similarity, she gets a sort of second hand unconscious passion directed toward only those qualities in which she resembles her mother-in-law (present or to be). In this type of man, any points of dissimilarity cannot be the objects of unconscious passion. So that a woman who has more dissimilarity from, than similarity to, the mother-in-law is perceived less as she is than as she is not. She exists for the man, only in her points of likeness to his mother. In her points of difference, she does not exist for him at all, nor can she exist, because of the screen, which is constantly and permanently before his eyes.

Sometimes a large part of her personality is thus completely screened out of existence as far as the man is concerned. For him only one per cent of her may exist at all, that proportion of similarity between herself and his mother. For a man who has not this permanent unconscious mental fixture, his wife is at least perceptible as she *is*, as far as his experience and culture enable him to see anything as it really is. But the man with the fixated mother imago, cannot remove it from his mental eye, and his wife cannot any more exist for him than if she were a head sticking through a steel partition, the rest of her being absolutely inaccessible. This is not only the explanation of why the mother-in-law cannot get on with the wife, but also why the man cannot really, because he cannot unconsciously, love, that is, feel passion for, his wife, and why he seeks prostitutes, or if not the professional prostitute, gives his love to one woman after another. He has been frustrated in his desires for his mother, somewhere between the ages of five and fourteen, and the disappointment, causing the repression of emotion, has been the cause of that particular desire being retained unchanged with that particular content. Frustrated in his first passion, he connects passion with frustration, in his unconscious mind, and now no object of it can satisfy it any better than the original one did. It is much as if he had been switched off the normal track, and could never get back on it again.

It might be supposed that if the mother had gratified the childish passion, this idea of frustration would not have become connected with it.

But there are legitimate ways in which the mother can gratify this passion without creating a fixation of it upon the mother imago formed at so early an age. And it might also be supposed, that if the passion were not originally directed toward the mother, it might be fortuitously directed toward some one else who also must have turned it back, so that if a man had not a mother imago, he might just as well have a first-love imago formed after the pattern of the first girl for whom he felt passion. And of course, we all know of men who have been disappointed in love and never able to love again.

D. *Unconscious Passion of Mother for Son*

The first steps in the direction of unconscious passion for mother are blocked by the mother herself, who, in diverting from herself the passionate current of her son's love, has no other direction in which to steer it. She generally attempts to stop it altogether, knowing that in the fourteen year old boy, there is in civilized society, no object available for it. She ought to tell the boy that if he has to kiss any one passionately, it should be some other woman, and of his own age; but no mother does this. If she were aware of any passionate element in the boy's kiss, she probably would tell him not to kiss her that way. But that the kiss is part affection and part passion, and that the passionate element may preponderate, even though it be unconscious, never seems to occur to the average mother.

Most mothers have an unconscious passion for their children. No one will deny that the act of suckling is rendered permanently a biological essential of motherhood, by virtue of its sensual, sexual feeling-reaction on the mother's part. Nor will any one believe that the passionate element of the mother's love for her son immediately vanishes at the time when the child is weaned from the breast, unless there is another child on the way toward being born. So that in this situation where the son is the only child, or the last one, there is likely to be a strong unconscious passion on the mother's part having this boy as object. The importance of this consideration is in the result it has upon her behaviour to this son. The passionate current in this mother unites with the affectionate current and makes her doubly anxious to be his slave. If she cannot, because he is her son, and too immature, satisfy her unconscious sensual cravings on him, she compensates for it with all the variety of actions to which the term affectionate is commonly, but erroneously applied.

And this kind of treatment reinforces the original affection the son felt for his mother, and draws in gradually the full force of his passion toward her, yet unconsciously, so that later, when he sees a girl who attracts him sexually, either of two results ensues. On the one hand, he is unable consciously, to transfer to her his passion, because he regards her consciously as of the same class as his mother, for whom, unconsciously, he feels passion. Affection, he can freely transfer to the young girl whom he regards as his potential wife, because there is no barrier placed by society upon this transfer. Affection may go where it lists, just because it does not necessarily draw passion after it. On the other hand, while he may unconsciously transfer his passion to the girl, he cannot consciously, because he has been brought up to believe that it is wrong to do so. And this produces in him a great conflict, varying in intensity, according to the strictness with which he has been enjoined from giving expression to passion in the presence of women of his own social level.

If under these circumstances he meets a girl of his own social level, who responds to his passionate acts, and opportunity arises such as that of the hail storm in Vergil's Æneid, he becomes Æneas to her Dido, and Rumour then begins her deadly work. Only eugenic reasons should then interpose any obstacle to their present union.

But if the girl, brought up as most girls are, rejects his advances, she does so on purely conventional grounds, which thereupon start a conflict in each of their souls. Now, if the boy has unconsciously and consciously transferred his passion to the girl, and this conflict arises, it is again only a matter of the strictness of his bringing up, what he does with his passion. He can try to satisfy it upon a woman of lower social level, thus reserving for the other girl only his affection and a part of his conscious passion, for the current called passionate, unlike the affectionate one, *tends* to preserve its own integrity, and, in this event, to go out entirely, that is conscious and unconscious together, toward the woman of the lower social level. At any rate, she represents to him *all* and not a part of his unconscious passion, but she may even attract to herself a bit of affection. The girl whom he loves, in the sense of feeling affection and conscious passion for her, gets only these, and, even if she would, can get from him none, or at most, only a part, of his unconscious passion. For passion is intense, extreme, extravagant, excessive, all-devouring, all-powerful, and stoops to no paltry refinements. The lower class woman will carry out with him all forms of sexual perversity, which, in one sense could never be called perversities, if they were carried out with a wife under circumstances of complete conscious and unconscious love, in conjunction with, or as preliminaries to, the perfect consummation. But with a woman with whom there can never be any idea of having a legitimate child, the extravagant expressions of passion become perversities only.

For this reason the man, whose wife does not love him both affectionately and passionately, will never get from her the complete catharsis of any of his emotions. Nor will he get it from prostitutes, for the affectionate component will either be lacking entirely or be present in only a small amount. Such a man on finding in his wife, a woman whose passion is blocked by unconscious inhibitions which prevent her from giving herself to him completely, is subject to a shock which is continually recurrent.

E. *The Normal Way*

But the normal way is for the unconscious passion to be first directed, not toward the mother, but toward some girl outside of the family, who can return this " calf " love, which is generally not destined to be final, because neither boy nor girl is fully developed, but which on the other hand, is not destined to create in the boy the pinning together of frustration and passion, which are always fastened together where the mother figures in the unconscious comedy.

As is pointed out by Mrs. Evans in her book,* the attitude of the mother, to the first outgoing of the boy's feelings toward some girl outside of the family, is an important factor in his development, and one in which the mother plays instinctively a harmful part, unless she has insight enough to counteract her own unconscious passion for her son. If she can listen to him as he praises a girl he has seen and not say disparaging words about the girl, or his feeling for her, she is acting wisely. The same holds true of the reaction of the father to the first manifestations of unconscious passion in his daughter for some young man, outside of the family. Instinctively he feels jealousy, which prompts him to make scathing remarks about the young man, or about young cubs in general, or about her premature feeling for them, all of these caused by his own unconscious passion for his daughter.

The mother's or father's encouragement of affection and discouragement of passion on the part of the boy for the mother, or sister type of girl, has a vital effect upon the love life of the man in wedlock. As the wife generally belongs to the mother-sister class, she suffers, in the man's unconscious, from the same incest barrier that applies to passion directed toward all the women of this class. The unconscious passion of such a

* Elida Evans: *The Problem of the Nervous Child*, N. Y., 1920, p. 73.

man may, therefore, be attached also to women of another class, where the incest barrier is not effective, while his conscious passion may be, generally is, properly directed toward the wife, with any additional amounts of affection of which he may be capable.

F. *Split in the Love Stream*

Some such men, as before indicated, in whom this split of the love stream into two currents, which have been turned in diverse directions by the accidental happenings of early youth, have been given an additional twist by the reaction to them of the mother. That these men are frequently quite unable to have children with their wives, while they can with other women, is a matter that is of vital importance to society, because it is one of the causes of prostitution and illegitimacy. Society, therefore, should take steps absolutely, to prevent the possibility of such a split taking place in the love life of the man. The only means available, is complete scientific instruction in the psychology, and not alone in the physiology of sex. The latter is definite and limited, and comparatively well understood. The former is the rock on which most marriages are wrecked. The psychology of sex is a recent science, and every discovery is of the utmost importance and value for the welfare of the individual. The fact that the love stream is under certain circumstances split in this way, is a discovery of recent sex psychology. The spreading of this knowledge is a pressing need on account of its relation to prostitution.

G. *Illicit Love*

No man will fail to see, if these facts are clearly presented to him, just what the significance of prostitution is. He will see that in seeking prostitutes, he is, in two senses, seeking his mother imago. In the first sense he is seeking in a woman not of his mother's class the gratification of unconscious desires for his mother, aroused by her in his childhood, and which she should not have been allowed to arouse, or should have been instructed how to gratify symbolically.

This is at one and the same time, a seeking and a turning from the mother imago. Unconsciously he seeks it to gratify what had been previously denied, because complete satisfaction can be got only from what was first desired and from no subsequent substitute. Consciously he seeks a woman *not* of the " mother " class, because of the conscious or fore-conscious inhibitions against any person of that class. In a second sense, he is seeking a replica of his mother imago, on whom to gratify his passion, because of the fact that his mother imago represents accessibility and easy compliance.

Thus are clearly represented, the two forms in which the mother imago may appear in the unconscious mind of the adult man. It is both compliant and inhibitive (or repellent) at the same time. The compliant phase of it he seeks in the woman, other than the wife, who belongs to the mother class, because the imago of the mother class woman contains the inhibition. The inhibition phase of it is transferred by him to all women of the mother class. It is of course, characteristically infantile to divide the world of women into only two classes—the mother class and the other class—but it is the case with many men.

A man, whose childish unconscious passion has been, by circumstances over which he has no control, unfortunately directed toward the women of his own family, is unlikely to be able to direct that passion to his wife. Unfortunately, he is generally unable to know this until after marriage.

H. *The Œdipus Situation*

The mother imago, once crystallized, the photographic negative of the mother, once fixed in the soul of the young man, has the double effect of determining his choice of an object for his unconscious passion and fastening it to the unconscious. What fastens it to the unconscious, and thus prevents its naturally coming into consciousness, is the fact that passion felt for mother is against nature, and in this type of man, passion has been felt for mother, through no fault of his own nor of his mother's, but through the force of circumstances which are as unknown to him, and until today as uncontrollable by him, as was the action, predestined by the fates, of Œdipus in marrying his own mother, Jocasta. In absolute ignorance of his real relation to her, he had four children of her. In absolute ignorance of his real relation to his mother imago, which is that of passion where affection only is natural, the modern man whom I am describing, marries not his own mother, but his mother imago. Just as the marriage of Œdipus and Jocasta caused misfortunes, whose origin was mysterious, to fall upon Thebes, so the always unsuccessful, and therefore continually repeated attempt of modern man to marry with his mother imago, has brought upon civilization the mysterious calamity of prostitution. And just as, in the Greek myth, the situation was illuminated by their science, the oracle, so, in our present age, the situation is being illuminated by our present oracle, scientific research.

Laius was killed by his own son Œdipus. By every male child, the father is killed in the mother's eyes, unless the proper insight be given to both father and mother. Though Œdipus was penetrating enough to solve the riddle of the Sphinx, he was not able to recognize even his own mother, because he had been taken away from her soon after birth. Therefore, instinct alone in humans is not enough to prevent inbreeding. For this reason science, the extension of consciousness over more and more of the external world, is necessary to raise man above the animals, and bring him to his fullest expression.

Possibly, too, the Œdipus myth contains an unconscious comment on the necessity of paying more attention to the very young. Œdipus, who was abandoned by his parents in his infancy, was the one who, therefore, could not remember his mother, and thus avoid marrying her. This is the unconscious criticism of the neglect, by the parents, of the intellectual and emotional life of their children. Engrossed in his regal duties, Laius heard only the oracle about the son to be born to kill him. In America we are all kings, and our children are killing us every day inasmuch as we are actually neglecting the real problem of developing out their utmost resources.

Let no one say, in reply to this, that he is sending his children to the best private schools, or that the public schools of the country are the best in the world in democratic spirit. It is true enough, but neither public or private schools have yet as much as faintly sensed the problem of the child's psychological relation to the parents within the family. No more has the parent realized that his relation to the child does not stop, when the child has been safely landed in a good school. In order to do the best for the child, the parent has to train himself to be a parent. In view of the great complexity of modern existence, it is no longer enough to give life to the child, and sustenance for a number of years. Many a man is quite proud of himself, because he likes children so well that he gives them more candy and peanuts than are good for them, or plays and romps with them every evening, or helps them with their Latin and Algebra, or oversees their getting a job that only his superior " pull " can get them. Such a man is not fit to be the father of a child in the psychological sense of a head of family that possesses power, but not too much, shows indulgence, but not too much, has care for the children, but not too much tenderness. And the same may be said of the mother. Unless she knows how to keep her hand off her children enough, and yet keep enough control over them, she is not fit psychologically to be a mother.

No one has yet taken any step worth mentioning, in the direction of the psychology of the family, to show parents just how their acts appear from the inside of the child's mind, and to show the parents how the inside of the child's mind really looks, and what they must do and not do, to secure the largest development of the child's powers. While many parents are so selfish as to wish their children not to be superior to them in any way, there are yet some who desire progress to be made in that direction. More time than they now give to golf and bridge, to reading fiction and to other relaxations, will have to be given by such people, to a thorough study of the psychological implications of:

1. a mother's having a daughter in the family
2. a mother's having a son in the family
3. a mother's having more than one son and daughter
4. a father's having more than one son and daughter
5. a father's having a daughter only
6. a father's having a son only

Every one of these six relations is subject to its peculiar risk, which is somewhat less if the family is larger, but still remains. The risk is psychological, not economic, except secondarily; not eugenic, not hygienic, primarily. The risk is to the psyche of the parent on the one hand, and to that of the child on the other.

No science of family life exists at the present time, other than that supplied by the researches of the modern psychologist into the nature and activities of the unconscious mind. Any part of familial living we may have at present is the result of chance trial and error method, determined itself largely by the interactions of the unconscious wishes of the two or more persons constituting the family. So wretched, too, has been the result of this fortuitous action, never yet taken up except by the almost despised sentiment of some good mothers, that families are in a spiritual condition not unlike armed neutrality, where petty jealousies reign controlled by the unconscious fears of inferiority, and by desires for personal aggrandizement.

This family-feud condition, which is only the uncultured reaction of the archaic unconscious to the total situation, might easily, and should quickly, be ameliorated. Grown-up brothers and sisters shrink from coming to an amicable understanding with each other, not to mention the resentments felt between parents and their grown-up children. I avoid the word adult, because it is to be kept for really adult reactions to the total situation. With the emotions aroused by this untutored arrangement of grown-up relatives, it is no wonder that politics is the mess it is, and that nations go to war with each other.

If parents would see to it that they themselves understood the manifold interactions of the condition of being husband, wife, father, brother, sister, son, daughter, etc., and insisted on their children being brought up in full knowledge of these relations and all they imply in the family, there would hardly be any need for politics in the nation, which would become what its name really signifies—community economics. But the ordinary person will say that a study such as I have indicated would take too much time and be too difficult. I admit that it would be difficult, and that it is the most difficult problem we have to face individually, but there is no problem so much worth the effort, because the results would be infinitely progressive, and would go farther than any other effort that men and women could make toward the securing of conditions, as different as could be, from the perfectly impossible conditions now obtaining in so-called civilization.

Civilization is based on the family and the relations of the members of the family to each other. The Œdipus myth represents so much of what is going on, not in the conscious life, but in the unconscious of the man of today, that it is interesting to note these few features of the story.

The ancient oracle said, that the man who had killed King Laius, Œdipus' father, must be found and punished. Modern science similarly says it is necessary to find and control the unseen power that has violated conjugal integrity. Science has shown that this person is no other than the child itself. He (or she), by appearing between the married pair, completes the original and inevitable triangle. The parents' ignorance of the effects of this total situation on the child is a part of the cause of the social evil, because the child, whether boy or girl, may grow up with a deeply fixated parent imago. Thus both parents and child are the cause, and, just on account of their ignorance, neither is responsible.

The photographic mental negative of the mother, or mother-imago screen, fixed in the soul of the man I am describing, prevents him from perceiving any woman at all. He cannot see her as she is; he cannot hear her voice as it really is; he cannot touch her for herself; he cannot spiritually appreciate her for what she really is, because in front of all his senses and his mental faculties stands the unchangeable representation of the mother person as she happened to be at the time this sensitive plate was exposed to her presence. This might seem to suggest that only those children who are more than ordinarily sensitive would so early receive and crystallize such an impression. This may indeed be the case, but their number is large. If they are young, they may be helped objectively by a change of environment, and, if they are older, they may be helped subjectively to gain conscious control over their unconscious passion and struggle free from a bond which is going to be permanently injurious.

A couple is said to fall in love with each other. They really should learn to rise to love each other. If Cupid is painted blind, because " love looks not with the eyes, but with the mind," this only means that Shakespeare knew the difference between conscious and unconscious passion. Here conscious passion is the eyes, and unconscious passion is the mind. Love cannot see with the eyes because of the blindness of the conscious passion to the very existence of the unconscious passion.

Any one will admit that he receives unconscious impressions from real objects, but is unwilling to grant that these form any considerable part of the motives of his actions, in spite of the facts that birds of a feather flock together, and that evil communications corrupt good manners. The blindness of love is only another way of expressing the idea that the individual is not aware of what unconscious love-desires prompt him in his wooing; or the blindness of love still

signifies that no one can directly see his own unconscious passion, which is nevertheless there,
even if he does not consciously make love.

Where it operates as a fixed photographic negative before the mental eye of the man, the mother
imago exists in its extreme form, but in all men
there are degrees of fixity, from absolute rigidity
to absolute fluidity. The socially approved degree is that which remains fluid until the individual marries, and then " sets " as adamant concrete hardens after a while. If the unconscious
passion of the soul sets too early, no woman will
fit the infinite requirements of it, simply because
no two humans are exactly alike and it requires
exact correspondence in the specifications of the
unconscious passion permanently to gratify its
desires. Then the man cannot ever still the universal longing of the soul for the perfect correspondence of a mate. But he is deceived over
and over again into thinking that he has found
her, because his great desires make him think
that a partial correspondence is a total one. It
is surprising and humiliating to him later to
find how a single one of the myriad qualities of
some woman has been seized upon by his unconscious passion and magnified, so that she seems
to him for a brief ecstatic moment to fulfil *all*
his requirements. But every later experience of
her shows him how small is the real correspon-

dence and how unable he is to change his own requirements.

If the unconscious passion of the soul " sets " too late, there will be a possibility that the man will be unable *not* to adapt himself to *any* woman who comes his way, and yields to him. In this he will be like the brutes, who have no greater specification than that their mates shall be of the same species as themselves. And there are, of course, many people like the brutes, who are satisfied if their mates be only human. But with these people we are not in this book concerned, except in so far as they might have it revealed to them that a complete respondence, caused by mutual adaptation each to other is an inestimable factor in promoting health and happiness, and, through these, efficiency and development,—results securable to the same degree by no other means.

I. *The Incest Barrier*

Too much emphasis cannot be laid upon the fact that the mother imago bears always in its outlines the inhibition of the incest barrier. The man seeing in a woman some insignificant similarity between her and his mother is completely swept off his feet by the fact of really finding what he has looked years to find, for it is a small chance that more than few women are bearers of this trait, whatever it is, who match even in one of the myriad qualities the pattern with which he is ever unconsciously comparing them.

A man, finding such a woman, immediately thinks his happiness is secured forever, tragically unaware of the fact that this responding trait will never be free from the taint of consanguinity, a trait that inexorably precludes his transferring to her, the sum total of his unconscious passion, because, on account of the inhibitions originating in the higher level of the fore-conscious, the unconscious passion cannot be felt for the real mother, or for any other woman indistinguishable from her. And the woman selected by the man with the unconscious mother imago will be indistinguishable unconsciously from the mother, no matter how clearly the man consciously sees that there are points of difference between them. His unconscious passion is blind to the differences and sees only the resemblances.

Therefore he will experience one disappointment after another in the woman whom he has married. His unquenchable desire has been trained to insatiability, by the very fact of having been repressed at an early age when repression is a black blight upon a tender bud. He is then practically forced to gain through a resort to other women the satisfaction of the desires prompted by his unconscious passion. And among the demi-monde he can find the gratification of his animal desires, because, removing himself from the operation of the civil law, he unconsciously regards himself as beyond the pale of natural law, too, and the incest barrier is no obstruction to him. With all women of his own social status, he would find unconscious passion blocked by the barrier made by their similarity to his mother.

If the passion of the man for his wife is the same kind in his unconscious as he has previously shown for his mother, he will be regarding his wife only as his mother, and the same sort of daily wrangling, as in the case of mother and son, mentioned elsewhere, will be continued. He will feel only unconscious passion for his wife, because she is only a substitute mother for him, and his conscious feelings will repeat the resentment and irritability, because his unconscious passion is fixated on his mother imago, to which it was originally attracted. Toward his wife he cannot express it consciously however, on account of the barrier society has set up against incest.

The incest barrier, which was the reason of his not being able consciously and overtly to feel and express passion for his mother, is still the same barrier between himself and his wife, who is reacted to, after a certain short time of married life, just as the mother was reacted to, after the boy experienced the rebuffs from her. If one's wife should suddenly be made known to one as his real mother, whom he had married without knowing who she really was, his mind would be filled with horror and pity. This is the fate, not only of the Œdipus of ancient Greek legend, but of many a man of the modern world who has married a woman who can be only a mother to him and not a real wife. She was chosen by a man's own unconscious passion which, fixated upon the mother imago, could not be fired by any other object than a woman visually or auditorially, or in some other sense quality like the mother. On the unconscious mind of a young man whose vision is so impeded or perverted by the ghostly lineaments of the negative made in the film of his child soul by the appearance and behaviour of his mother at her most blooming age, no girl makes any impression except in so far as she resembles his mother's character portrait, carried in the living tissues of his brain; and any girl's effect upon him is great, if she closely resembles in form or character, the image he unconsciously worships, though he may despise the personality of his mother at the present time. Love at first sight is of so complete and sudden a character as to indicate at once that the unconscious passion has instantly fastened itself upon the personality of some young replica of the former, but not now existing, woman. And love at first sight has the compulsive character which one would naturally expect in a passion which has been fixated—crystallized so as to react only in certain definite and unchanging ways.

If there were two women in the world so exactly alike that this man's actual flesh and blood wife could be, by any test, quite indistinguishable from the mother imago (or the real mother, thirty years ago), it would seem that then the unconscious passion of the man could be fixated upon the younger woman. But, even so, the unconscious passion toward the mother must remain unconscious. It has been rendered unconscious by repression at the hands of the real mother. By the real mother it has been repressed only on account of the incestuous nature of such a relation. The unconscious passion for the actual wife is still repressed, because she is to all intents and purposes his mother. It would be as " wrong " for him to love the one, as it would be to love the other, in a passionate way. And the bringing into consciousness of the unconscious passion is the only means by which a man can truly come perfectly and wholly to love his wife. So that if the man with the fixated mother

imago, succeeds in bringing into consciousness
the unconscious passion for his wife, he will find
that it is really an incestuous passion for his
mother, while more of the qualities in the woman,
which have unconsciously been picked out by the
man in conformity with his mother imago, are
unlike the mother imago, than like it, such a man
is carried away by finding a woman with some
few characteristices like his mother ideal.   In
his imagination he emphasizes these likenesses
and naturally overlooks, for he is constitutionally
unable to see, in the ardour of his first infatua-
tion, the qualities in the real young woman that
are dissimilar to his ideal of a woman formed in
him in his childhood.   But later, when he has
more intimate acquaintance with her, and should
be able to see her more nearly as she really
is, he would be expected to transfer his unconscious passion gradually to her bit by bit, and
finally accept her altogether as she is, and not as
he first idealized her.   And if she is a healthy and
wholesome young woman, the progressive revelation of her peculiar characteristics should have
an exciting and alluring effect upon his unconscious, as well as upon his conscious, passion.

That is, however, the case of the absolutely
normal man, with no unconscious fixation of passion upon an entirely imaginary person.   And,
for the kind of man I am now describing, this

woman he has married, is an absolutely imaginary person, who is expected to act in ways quite in accordance with a preconceived notion, determined by the man's own experience of his mother, when he was one to five years old, and she anywhere from sixteen to forty-five. For such a man, the disappointments are innumerable, and inevitable. His unconscious passion is moulded in such a way, as to be adaptable only to a woman in all respects exactly like his mother when he was a child. His expectations are absolutely definite, and constitute a list of specifications as elaborate as those for the construction, from the foundation to flag-staff on the topmost tower, of a forty-story office building— specifications with which no living woman could possibly comply, as they are not only derived from a woman no longer existent, but also added to and complicated by the experience and phantasies of the man himself.

By such a man every action of his wife is scrutinized, even though unconsciously, for its minute correspondence with these complicated specifications, and every deviation from them is measured and compiled and collated into a group of disappointments, resentments and hates which accumulates from hour to hour, and day by day.

J. *The Crystallized Man*

In order for a man to get pleasure from a life-long association with a woman, his psyche should be elastic and adaptable, and capable of experiencing joy from surprises, and unexpected revelations in the character of his wife, but the man I have been describing, has a fixated and not a free unconscious passion. The surprises are endless, but all give displeasure rather than pleasure, for he is crystallized before his time. He is an aged soul in a young body.

The result of his unconscious crystallization is a plurality of women. This he manages to accomplish in an infinite number of ways. Prostitution is only one of them, including, as they do, intimacies of various degrees, from purely intellectual, Platonic devotion to, and attendance upon, some other woman than his wife, down to illicit sex relations of any degree of grossness. But they are all caused by the fact that his unconscious passion, being fixated upon an imago, is unable, because of its inexorably unchangeable nature, to find complete satisfaction in any living woman. Therefore, he runs from one to another, sometimes very rapidly, and he must continue to keep running, because he is destined never to find a real woman who can fulfil all his requirements.

No such woman exists. One might believe that, if the women, whom such a man tries on, fully realized that they were all being merely tried on, to see if they would fit an imaginary dummy in the man's distracted mind, they would see the impossibility of their position and would give him no encouragement. But the majority of such women are in exactly the same predicament as the men. Having crystallized specifications in their own unconscious passion, due to a father or brother imago, they are in their turn only trying on one man after another, in the really hopeless search for a real man to fit an imaginary dummy in their own souls.

As there are not two women who look and act exactly alike, the chance does not exist that a man will find in a woman the exact duplicate of his mother, and, on longer intimacy with her, he will find more and more traits in which she deviates from his mother imago. These differences will first puzzle, then annoy, and finally estrange him unconsciously, even though he consciously thinks her the best and most wonderful woman in the world.

It might appear that the more she deviated from the mother imago, the more he could feel unconscious passion for her, just because of the absence of the incest barrier, and that the unconscious barrier might then unite with the conscious passion and complete a perfect love. But it must be remembered that the complete love, which is the combination of conscious and unconscious passion, must be freely directed to one woman, and that, in the man with the fixated unconscious passion (fixated, I mean, upon the mother imago), there is ever present the incest barrier, which is a barrier against *any* direct expression of unconscious passion in the presence of any woman of the mother class. In other words, the fixated unconscious passion can never become conscious, because it *is* fixated, and, as it can never become conscious, it cannot become free to attach itself to the deviations or the deviating elements, even in the wife who is seen first unconsciously as a mother, and later is unconsciously realized as differing more and more from the mother imago. In this sense, the more a woman of the mother class *differs* from this fixated mother imago of the man, the *less* will he be able to feel unconscious passion for her, the less appeal will she have for his personality below the threshold.

K. *Passion Indispensable*

It is unquestionable that not only should the wife be the object both of the affection and the passion of the husband but that the husband should be the object of both the conscious and the unconscious passion of the wife. But it frequently happens that the same split in the love stream of the woman herself has taken place, because of circumstances analogous to those obtaining in the case of the man. She is unduly impressed, though quite unconsciously, by the personality of her father, and, with men of the father-brother class, associates affection only. The same incest barrier is opposed to the first manifestations of her unconscious passion, which she naturally directs toward the man or men of her family. Girls especially suffer from this repression, and chiefly because they do not break through the inhibitions against sex expression laid down by society. In addition to this they are affected retroactively by the conduct of men of the father-brother class themselves. Therefore there exists this double cause for the large proportion of anesthetic women, or women whose passion is only unconscious, a condition which alone may cause some men otherwise normal to resort to prostitution.

With regard to the comparative status of affection and passion the attitude of individual members of society toward passion varies. It is conventionally accepted that affection may be openly expressed for people of both sexes, for animals and for things, but there is, in the minds of those people who are brought up with ignorant notions about sex, the idea that passion is something brutal, sensual, reprehensible, degrading. The heavenly love, which is affection, and the earthly love, which is passion are contrasted, and the feelings of exhaustion and depression experienced by some people after gratification of the sensual passion are regarded as marks of its lower na‧ ture. This causes a motive in some people to repress this part of their vitality. But these feelings of depression are not normal, and are only the result of indulgence by persons whose psyche is the seat of a conflict. For various reasons they can express their passion only fragmentarily. The bad feelings come only from the broken psyche causing the body to function without unity. Due to the splitting of the body by psychic inhibitions in the most intimate marital relations there is a racking effect never intended by Nature.

This leads to an erroneous judgment about passion on the part of many persons. As the results with them are unsatisfactory, they infer that there is some guilt connected with these activities. And certain ones, both men and women, come to the conclusion that passion is neither necessary nor wholesome. Women whose psyche is thus split make the demand that their husbands be satisfied with affection, which is a

physical impossibility unless the passionate current be successfully sublimated; and in marriage,
with intimate living together, it is neither possible nor desirable to sublimate all of it. The
wedded pair consisting of a passionate man on
the one hand and on the other a woman whose
conscious passion is directed toward her husband, but whose unconscious passion is repressed
for any reason, constitutes a breeding place for
unhappiness unequalled anywhere else in the
world.

L. *Prostitution from the Man's Standpoint* *

It may seem that the prostitute cannot be regarded as a mother imago, if she is the female
to whom the mother imago has driven the man,
or if the mother imago has been the only barrier
against the man's complete transfer to a wife.
From the old viewpoint the prostitute has been
the bulwark protecting the lawful wife from the
grosser sensuality of the husband, but the new
point of view is that she attracts to herself one
of the components of lawful married love—unconscious passion—and makes it difficult for
many, and impossible for some, to transfer their
entire love to their wives. The diversion of this

* In section F of the next chapter I shall have something
more to say about a possible aspect of prostitution from the
woman's standpoint.

component from its socially destined end to an asocial end not only constitutes a cause for a large proportion of professional prostitution, but it also results in dividing the man against himself; for the passionate component, which is the one that is free from fixation on the mother imago, makes him a man'out of a child, is much the more intense and is devoted to the race-perpetuating instinct, which in prostitution is subordinated to the autoerotic. When on the other hand the man seeks his mother imago in the prostitute, he is both autoerotic and unconsciously incestuous. The incestuous seeking of the mother imago belongs more to an asexual type of reproduction, as in budding, while the exogamous choice of a mate is a sexual reproduction of a higher type. We thus have prostitution from the male point of view regarded from two angles, from one of which it appears that in prostitution the man is unconsciously seeking an incestuous relation, in looking for the mother type of woman. From the other angle it appears that the man is unable to transfer the affectionate element of the love life to the woman who satisfies the desires arising from the sensual or passionate element.

This brings into clear view the conscious and social nature of affection, as contrasted with passion. Passion may normally attach itself to any member of the opposite sex, and normally does at least react to attractive members of the other sex unconsciously, even if it does not consciously do so. Affection is entirely determined by conscious factors, and by only such factors of the total situation as are consciously perceived; and, as we have seen, they are few in number compared with the unconscious factors. Also affection is that amount of feeling which is stirred by a conscious knowledge of social relations. Passion is the feeling stirred by concrete qualities of persons only, not merely those consciously perceived but by the much greater number of personal qualities unconsciously perceived, and by the trends and tendencies integrated by former concrete experiences.

If a man were able to transfer his affection to a woman outside of the pale of social respectability, he would have to dispose of all his ideas consciously acquired from contact with his family,— ideas which, in his fore-conscious, have been integrated into a code of morality containing modes of emotional reaction antipathetic to women of loose morals. If he were able to transfer his affection to such women, he would himself remain a unity.* Psychologically he might then be the real husband of an unreal wife.

---

* See discussion of erotic unity and disintegration in section H of the next chapter.

M. *Real Husband of Unreal Wife*

Being the real husband of an unreal wife, the animate husband of an inanimate wife, the intact husband of a fragmentary wife, the hundred per cent husband of a one per cent wife, the feeling husband of an unfeeling wife, is exactly what any man is unconsciously trying to be to any prostitute, if he is capable of transferring to her his entire conscious and unconscious passion. But he will never succeed in being completely real, for he will never be able to deliver his affection to the same destination. The very fact that she is looked down upon by society will divide his affection from his passion, and his love life is but rent in twain, if he cannot direct both to the same woman.

Being the real wife of an unreal husband, the feeling wife of an unfeeling husband, is what we hear of most frequently, and what we generally expect to hear, because of a universal notion that women are more susceptible to the finer emotions, and are as a whole more emotional than men. The truth is that men are equally emotional, but that they are so brought up as to have more insight into their sexual life than do women. They can more frequently become real husbands, whether of real or of unreal wives, because their unconscious passion is more generally revealed to them than is that of women.

Even to his real wife an unreal husband transfers his affection successfully, and she therefore would become a mother imago to him, and in this would be an incestuous object, if the object of affection could be called incestuous; but it is only the object of passion that can be so called. The transfer of passion to the mother is the original and universal incestuous relation referred to in the Œdipus myth. The sub-human instinct would be to transfer the passion to the nearest female as soon as passion began. Human society with its incest barrier prohibits only this transfer, having no prohibition against the direction of affection toward any person, animal or thing. Unconsciously, in the human man-child, passion becomes transferred to the incestuous object and remains fixated there while consciously there is an inhibition against the transfer of passion to the incestuous object. This is the earliest and commonest conflict in the psyche.

The possible combinations of conscious and unconscious passion on one side or other, directed toward the other, with or without response, are very numerous. There are over a thousand such combinations, if we include also the presence or absence of insight in one or other or both of the pair, and the factor of mutuality, and out of them there can be only one form of absolutely happy marriage, that in which both conscious and unconscious passion of both is directed each toward the unconscious passion of the other, and in which both have insight. It will be necessary therefore to explain a little in detail what is meant by insight.

CHAPTER IV

A. *Thinking of Things Together*

SOME people cannot as quickly as others recognize and name a piece of music that they hear. They feel that the music is familiar, but they cannot recall what it is, nor what is associated with it. A connection fails to be made between the name of the piece or that of the composer and the sounds themselves. This is analogous to the lack of insight in conscious and unconscious passion. There the connection fails to be made between the one and the other. The unconscious passion nevertheless exists, and is the sounding board over which the pretty tune of the emotions is played, but the individual fails to name it correctly, sometimes even if he has been told again and again. There is evident a strong unconscious wish either to banish the name, or to disconnect the name with the feelings. " This means you " is needed to be emphasized repeatedly. *De te Fabula narratur.*

This brings out an important peculiarity about insight. It is always endogenous. It never can be given. There are none so blind as those that do not wish to see. Therefore experience can be the only successful teacher, and statements learned by rote avail nothing. The aim of the higher education, namely bringing out what is within, is therefore attained mostly by indirect means,— by bringing together the name and the music and hoping the connection between them will be sensed. This aim is the more clearly recognized nowadays than ever before, and particularly in the recreation movement, where the unconscious passion's manifestations are being enlisted.

Telling any one directly that his acts are an expression of unconscious passion always tends to evoke the same antagonism that is called forth by telling him anything else, except the merest matter of fact information asked for, such as what day of the month it is or what hour of the day. The most " telling " things are situations in which the individual cannot fail to see how he stands, and all that education, of whatever sort, can do is artfully to bring about these situations in such a way as to provoke the inevitable and instinctive unconscious response. If this reaction is frequent and emphatic enough, the individual will finally " see " the implications of his thought and actions.

B. *The Adumbration*

A peculiar and characteristic feeling marks the approach of some ideas into consciousness. It is caused by the wish of the idea which is in the unconscious to enter into the light of consciousness. The quick succession of ideas in the case of wit is an example that is attended by great buoyancy and exuberance of spirits. I do not here refer particularly however to that type of phenomena, but to that which is much more available for scientific study—the slow and halting occurrence of an idea that is foreshadowed by many indefinite, almost indescribable, feelings. It is quite a different feeling from the conscious desire to recall something, a name for example. At a big dance a young man was introduced to Miss Black, a very beautiful girl. He danced with her a few minutes and found her most agreeable. A little later a man friend of his asked who she was and wanted an introduction. He looked around and, seeing what he thought was the same girl, took his friend up to her and said: " Miss Black, let me introduce Mr. Brown." Something in the situation gave him the peculiar familiar feeling, but, as in most such occasions, he could not make it definite enough to know exactly what it meant. Afterward he wondered if he had introduced his friend to the wrong girl. So he asked some one else and found out that he had taken his friend to Miss Green and called her Black to her face.

One sometimes goes into a room and forgets what one has gone there for, or to a bookshelf for a certain book and forgets what book one went for. The state of mind in these situations is quite similar to the feeling experienced, sometimes on starting out from home, that we have forgotten something. It is a feeling of uneasiness or dissatisfaction which, if not attended to, may soon pass away. When later we realize what we have forgotten, e. g. a letter that we meant to post, we wonder why we did not heed the warning given us by the unconscious, which took in the whole situation of the circumstances of the departure. The disappointment felt later with so much greater intensity is no proof that the indefinite emotion was not existent in the unconscious both before and after it made its temporary appearance in consciousness.

These states of mind may be called adumbrations of an approaching idea—a foreshadowing in which only the proximity of something is indistinctly sensed, without any definiteness or clear lineaments. Occasionally, as in the going into a room for something, or to a bookshelf for some book, the situation is definitely relieved, if the object is thought of. Then one knows that *that* was what was foreshadowed. In this respect it is something resembling the mental search for a name, but yet there is a difference.

The adumbration in the case of the approach of unconscious passion is generally however not so much a state of mind, but it is very definite and concrete group or series of acts. Without any psychic adumbration entering his consciousness, the boy of fourteen will give some girl of sixteen a present. He does not of course recognize it as a mark of his unconscious passion for her. There is a goodly vocabulary of terms by means of which to euphemize his feeling, from "attention" through "interest" to "fascination."

In the very young the unconscious passion has a direct pathway from the unconscious to a concrete act. A girl of two years and six months was playing in the country under the trees before the piazza and said to a little three-year-old boy, " Jimmie, I want to kiss you." Jimmie nonchalantly accepted the kiss. The unconscious passion of the little girl found a direct path not only to acts but to words. There could not be said to be any conscious passion in her act. It was purely instinctive. Later on the present of the youth to the maiden is a symbolical kiss, also a mark of unconscious passion.

It should be remembered that much of what is *called* affection is really the unrecognized conscious manifestation of unconscious passion. In the strictly scientific sense the term affection should not be applied to any love felt by one sex toward the other, if it is possible to interpret it as unconscious passion.

C. *Insight*

By insight is meant therefore man's or woman's ability to see that the actions of conscious passion are the result of the unconscious passion and to make due allowances therefor. Ellen Key * says: "The senses go their own way and are attracted where the soul is estranged, or repelled although the heart is filled with tenderness. Until the physiology and psychology of loathing are understood, we shall not have gone far toward the solution of the erotic problem. Every day—and night—these innumerable influences, conscious or unconscious, are at work transforming the feelings of married people and

* This and the following two quotations from Ellen Key are a good illustration of the defects of such writers. They fail to analyze completely and examine minutely and correlate adequately. Analysis has shown how to interpret, and so to control, the "important trifles of married life." In saying that "man's senses are spurred by a desire which thrusts aside that of the soul" the writer quoted fails to realize the enormous effect of the soul—by which she means social and intellectual life—in curbing man's senses to the permanent detriment of man as a whole. (See Chap. V, Sec. E.) She fails, too, in mentioning the mysterious effects of elective affinities, to take account of the very definite results of analytical psychology in removing the mystery and explaining just what these elective affinities are.

lovers. And although our time is becoming increasingly conscious of this, it does not yet understand how to counteract the dangerous or encourage the favourable influence of the important trifles of married life." This ability to understand the relation between the conscious and unconscious passion will in the future be directly in proportion to the amount of real information possessed, the amount of scientific knowledge imparted in childhood by the proper persons.

In literature we find illustrations of all types of conscious and unconscious passion described. Miranda is made a woman without insight falling in love with a man having insight. Nahum Tate rehashed Shakespeare's *Tempest* so that both Miranda and Ferdinand should show lack of insight.

Phyllis and Corydon wander through the glades without insight. In modern times Jack and Jennie, aged fourteen and twelve, stroll in the gloaming attracted by each other. They kiss to the accompaniment of mysterious feelings, indefinite and shimmering, which neither of them understands. Every touch of palm to palm, or palm to shapely waist is an invitation to further experience, but neither knows what the feelings signify. Each look that is so full of emotion is quite as empty of definite meaning. This is the eternal call of unconscious passion to unconscious passion. " Meanwhile mankind continues to be guided by erotic impulses which lie deep below its conscious erotic needs. Man's senses are spurred by a desire which thrusts aside that of the soul " (*Ib.* p. 72). " Every human being who himself has soul is being more and more penetrated by the sense of the mysterious effects of elective affinities; of sympathetic and antipathetic influences; of subconscious powers, above all in the erotic sphere " (*Ib.,* p. 82). Following the instincts prompted by the call of unconscious passion the young people would inevitably unite as Nature intended them to do. Above this figured bass of unconscious passion runs a pretty melody which captivates the young people and makes them consciously long to be together, but there are yet to be added the intermediate voices of the harmony, the knowledge not alone of the physiology of the emotion but also of the social relations yet to be unfolded in the mutual lives of the two.

When they know the poem of love from beginning to end, and of the life which will spring from their lives, they will see in every line of it the reference to the reciprocal love of their two lives. This is when every incident of every day has a double significance because it is to be reflected in the mirror of the other soul. The mannerisms of other men and women, their deeds and their peccadilloes, their likes and dislikes, will all be related to the main current of life which is love, as never they were before, and the existence of other men and women striving blindly or with insight, becomes a source of unending interest to lovers, who see in others the replica of themselves, wherein they rejoice with an exceeding joy, or they see a pair less fortunate and they grieve for them only by trying to give them help or light on their situation, which is the best kind of help. And as will be seen, the insight of two people of opposite sex may be perfect or fragmentary, or may not be at all, so that in the various ways in which insight may be present in one or another or both of a pair, may have a great effect upon their happiness, for happiness comes from understanding and understanding from just this insight into the relation between conscious and unconscious passion.

The revealing of an unconscious passion is the emergence of that passion or sum of unconscious desires, from the unconscious into consciousness. The moments in which a man becomes conscious of desires in himself which had formerly been unconscious are moments in which there is a strong emotional reaction of surprise, pleasure and power. In such moments a man sees a great flash of light which makes relations visible that were invisible before, and shows him the connections between his acts and his thoughts, or between his acts and those of other people—connections whose invisibility had previously left the world of human behaviour bizarre, mechanically kaleidoscopic and unaccountable. He sees why most people regard marriage as a lottery in which there are ten thousand blanks to one prize. He sees too how it may be possible in the future to prevent marriage from being a lottery and to make it a work of art, the mutual work of both of the parties.

D. *Marriage as a Lottery*

Regarding marriage as a lottery is the childish attitude of people who seek to reject rather than to ameliorate necessary conditions found to be unpleasant. It is the attitude of the child toward the mother, which is that of the gambler toward Dame Fortune. As in the ignorant view of marriage, the view of those who regard it as all chance, the gambler expects from the minutest physical and mental effort on his part to gain the greatest material and emotional return, just as the very young child expects, quite normally and naturally, to receive everything from the mother and to render no return in action. " Can you not love me for what I am rather than for what I do? " is the question each one of some married pairs ask the other from time to time. But this is a question to which only a child could rationally expect an affirmative answer.

This fatalistic attitude is well illustrated by that of delinquent girls described by Maud E. Miner: * "The runaway girl is usually on the way to prostitution. . . . Under pressure of conditions at home, with discouragement and unhappiness, she throws all to the winds and plunges ahead into the dark. She sees nothing but her own troubles and does not care what happens. There is an element of curiosity in it too. Somewhere just a little further on, when free from the bonds of home and parents, she vaguely expects a world of happiness. In the blindness of ignorance or love she takes the first step, and then discovers that the sentence passed upon her by society is so severe that it is hard for her to return."

The blindness of love is the lack of insight on the young girl's part, or in some cases on the part of the young man, and insight is frequently if not always the result of wholesome enlightenment on sex matters. The blindness of love is the animal instinct which in humans has been inherited as unconscious passion. Humans have taken into consciousness so much that was in-

* *Slavery of Prostitution, A Plea for Emancipation*, N. Y., 1916.

stinctive in animal life, the rearing of children
and the building of homes and all the network of
modern social existence. They are now beginning to take into consciousness much more of the
mating instinct than ever they did before. The
taking of things into consciousness instead of
leaving them in the unconscious is a distinctive
mark of humanity, and the human activities last
taken into consciousness are naturally the oldest
and most fundamental, namely the love instincts.
In doing this they depart most widely from the
brute, for only humans exercise the mating instinct consciously and for other purposes than
for reproduction of young.

In fact the reproduction of young takes in
the average woman less than ten per cent of her
life time and in the average man an amount of
time so short as to be absolutely negligible. Any
time spent by the man in consciously practising
the actions suggested by the love instinct is almost exclusively taken up in the details of amplifying it, controlling it, and sublimating its
components into the organized factors of modern
society.

He spends more time in amplifying it, for
alone of all the animals he knows the meaning of
heredity and the permutations of elements composing it. Man alone has been able to idealize
sex, and to see that it is the moving force, the

spark which vitalizes so much more of inanimate matter directly and indirectly today than ever before. Man alone has made love out of the animal mating instinct, has made it cover more and more of human activity, so that now every atom of the social fabric is an expression of either perfect or perverted love.

One should not however forget that some men and women are much farther advanced in their insight into the mating instinct than are others, and that the control of the number of offspring is practised by them with full consciousness of what it implies for themselves and for society, and that without infanticide, abortion or ascetic abstinence. The practice of contraception is the most conscious thing man has done in his progress upward from the brutes. Taking control of that instinct which has been either uncontrolled by most, or repressed by a few men, mankind has now shown how it is not only possible but desirable and altogether sane, wholesome and hygienic to gratify the desires of conscious and unconscious passion. And latest of all he has shown that conscious and unconscious passion have long been separated in quite a considerable proportion of civilized men and women, due primarily to their civilization itself. And, best of all, that knowledge has begun to shed a ray of light on the most ancient ill of all society, prostitution, demonstrating that a new kind of marriage is possible in which, because of scientifically understood human mating, there could be no thought on the man's part of dissatisfaction or of infidelity to the monogamic principle, a principle that has been foreshadowed by the sexual relations of many animals and which man has most perverted in polygamy, polyandry, concubinage and prostitution.

E. *Affection and Both Passions Necessary*

So we can now say to all young people, and it is our duty to say it as emphatically as it can be said: Your love is composed of affection and of passion. Affection may be bestowed on all persons and things, for it is the connective tissue of society, and the basis of the surely coming brotherhood of all men. But your passion, if you are a man, is to be reserved for one woman, and for one man, if you are a woman, and you must learn to understand and realize the fact that while affection is entirely a conscious matter, passion is both conscious and unconscious. If you are not conscious of any passion, it means not that you have no passion, but that what you have is hidden from you. It is manifesting itself in many, if not all, of your acts and in the general trend of your behaviour. If you do not recognize it as passion, it is because you have not been as much enlightened as you should be. If you recognize it as passion and fail to see its relations to your family, and to your friends and fellow-citizens, you are still insufficiently enlightened. You will later learn, then, that not only does the knowledge of conscious and unconscious passion and the control and proper alignment of both, make you better citizens, but it makes you an asset to the community rather than a liability, because it maintains your bodily health. Your perfectly rounded individuality cannot exclude your body. No more can it exclude the normal functions of all your bodily organism, which include the relaxations of tensions set up in your involuntary muscles all over your body by the operation of your sympathetic or vegetative nervous system. In fact it has recently been shown that the voluntary muscles have been evolved for the sole purpose of ministering to the needs of the organism of involuntary muscles within them, which carry on all the physiological processes taking place within you. Your mentality is absolutely conditioned by the properly proportioned exercise of both voluntary and involuntary muscles. Your ability to think creatively is dependent upon your creative use of your body, which does not only imply procreating children, but does imply the conscious modification of the original animal mating instinct in such a way as to be buoyantly happy and cheerful all the time. No work of your hands or brains, no matter how seemingly remote from conscious or unconscious passion, is uninfluenced by both.

F. *Woman without Insight*

In chapter II, section B, " A Woman's Unconscious Passion," I have given an example of an "innocent" woman without insight. Her ignoring, whether conscious or unconscious, of the social significance of the relations of her acts resulted in her blinding herself to the harm she might be doing to the young men for whom she played adorable mother. But the woman without insight, whether this be dulled by use or never existent, is frequently likely either to become one of loose morals or, in any case, surely destined to become a potential if not an actual demi-mondaine. On the other hand, no woman with perfect love united of affection, conscious and unconscious passion and insight, can potentially approach the condition of looseness. Her feelings are all attached to the same man, and the right man, and her devotion is complete and final. In her we have not Griselda, whose fidelity is unreasoning, but Imogen (Cymbeline), whose love is flawless and supernal.

In one respect, therefore, the wife without insight is on the same sexual grade as the prostitute, who offers her conscious passion to the
passer by on the street for pay. The prostitute
has learned to direct her conscious passion for
the time being now to one and now to another
strange man, but her unconscious passion is not
thereby enlisted. Forcibly repressing all emotions of disgust and repulsion, which are consequently redoubled in force in her unconscious,
and cause a racking of the whole psychophysical
mechanism down to the postural tonus of the
muscles of every internal organ of her body, she
creates in herself a tension that can only be
relaxed by the extravagant brutality of her
" lover " or " bully," to whom she transfers both
conscious and unconscious passion.

But the wife with a fixated father imago, and
lacking insight, does practically the same thing
to her husband as the prostitute does to her
patrons and is no better off biologically or psychologically. Ignorant of the diverted trends of
her conscious and unconscious passion, and yet
not to blame for *her* ignorance any more than is
the prostitute to blame for not knowing what she
does, the wife submits to the embraces of her
lawful husband with the same unconscious racking. Like the prostitute she has learned to direct
her conscious passion but not to control her un-

conscious passion, and the two point different
ways. The result is as successful and scientific
as would be the attempt to fly an aeroplane, one
or two of whose four propellers revolved in opposite directions from the others.

The question naturally comes up how best to
secure insight in the woman as well as in the
man. As above suggested the only way is by
means of imparting in a matter of fact manner,
the scientific knowledge about the physiology,
and particularly about the psychology, of sex.
The chief contribution of science to psychology
has been just this recognition of the existence
and activity of the unconscious mental processes.
The unconscious desire is a desire for certain
gratifications that can be attained by conscious
movements of the body. But conscious movements are conscious in two senses. They may
be involuntary movements of which one later
becomes conscious that one has made them, or
they may be voluntary movements which are pic-
tured in imagination before they are carried out
in reality. Now in the person without insight
the conscious movements of the body which facili-
tate or render possible the gratification of the
unconscious desires are conscious only in the first
sense, namely, that they are so-called involuntary
movements of which one becomes conscious after
they are made.

Examples of involuntary actions manifesting unconscious passion have been given in the first chapter. They are observable by persons with insight in those without insight every day of the year. The man who has insight and is courting a girl that is deficient in insight will take advantage of his superiority in this ability and hugely enjoy the procedure. Many of the stories in Boccaccio's *Decameron* are of just this situation. Indeed it used to be the fashion carefully to bring up girls without insight, just because of this delight afforded men by the sense of superiority and power produced by this particular quality of maidenhood.

But the modern feminist movement is a movement for insight in women.

G. *The Vicious Circle*

Unconsciously men do not want prostitution to stop, because they want the mother-infant relation produced indefinitely. They want the mother-infant situation reproduced in their own love lives because they have not themselves been weaned psychically. They have not been spiritually weaned because their own mothers have not known how to do it. Their mothers have not learned to wean them spiritually because they have been brought up mental infants themselves. They have been kept mental infants by men, and there we have completed the vicious circle, in which the ultimate cause of irregular sex relations is the mother herself—model of sexlessness and paragon of purity.

But due to the never-ending power of truth to illuminate gradually more and more of human behaviour, a power that is now perverted, now wholesomely directed, by the periodical press, the drama and other means of communication, the vicious circle is being broken in many places, and insight, like freedom to a long term prisoner, is being forced upon women, and woman, formerly unenlightened, is now in the fight to enlighten men by giving insight to her sisters to prevent them from being man's involuntary and unwitting nursing bottles.

H. *Unity of Passion*

It is thus evident that a man may destroy the unity of his own passion. He may repress his desires for the body of his fiancée, and take the body of some other woman. Or, without going so far as to do this kind of splitting, he may be conscious of passionate desires for his affianced, and may repress or control them. He may carefully arrange his meetings with her so as not to allow himself any chance to give expression to his passionate desires. Or he may walk in the woods with her and kiss and fondle her. Different men stop at different stages on the path from mere affection to complete union, halted by less or greater sensitivity to the demands society makes upon them.

The implication in a novel like *Scandal* by Cosmo Hamilton is that a young woman of the social level of Beatrix Vanderdyke going with an artist into his studio at midnight is not stopping at any stage on the above path. A lack of internal control in both man and woman is implied by the strictness of the external bulwark. Or possibly it is unconsciously intended to denote that the persons, who are so circumscribed by conventions, need to be so, because they are so highly bred, like a fine strain of animals, who, once they got started, would brook no impediment to the satisfactions of their desires.

But in any case the inhibition exists, whether it be internal or external, and it does or does not break down, according to circumstances, or if it does not break down, it weakens at one point or another. The important consideration is the internal inhibition and the effect it produces in the physiological activities of the body.

The young man may not be conscious of any passion for the girl he likes. He may be conscious of the fact that he has no passion for her. But this is a fact of the conscious life alone. Its opposite is generally true of his unconscious. Otherwise he may belong in that class of men whose unconscious passion is permanently directed toward the mother imago. He likes the girl, feels affection for her, is interested in what she says and does, enjoys being with her, but never strongly desires to touch her. His affection easily passes from one girl to another, and sometimes he courts one of them in a mild way with respectful attentions, but no fire, until she is snapped up by some more lusty man. He then becomes her friend or her dog, and remains unsexed. There is no proof that his passion is less than that of his successful rival. The rival's passion is free to seek whom it will, his own passion is bound, in incestuous fixation upon his mother imago. The unconscious passion of these men who are unsuccessful wooers for the high type of women like their mothers, is still fixated upon the mother imago, which in this case is of the mild, complacent type. They find in the easy compliance of the demi-mondaine, the yielding quality they have missed in the proud ladies they have sought in vain.

Sometimes even these men succeed by chance in marrying their choice. If such a man does, he finds his wife after marriage as inaccessible as before, because of her unconscious perception that he is merely a child seeking a mother. This implies that in this instance the man is lacking in insight. He does not realize the similarity between the demands he makes on his wife to give him pleasure of various kinds and the demands made by a young child upon his mother. The wife unconsciously observes the several elements of this situation, and, even though she is not aware of them severally, she is quite aware of the dissatisfaction she feels in his love.

I. *Erotic Disintegration*

Erotic unity is a term that might be applied to the conscious and unconscious passion, when they are united by insight. Erotic disintegration is the condition of the man who thinks he can satisfy, or that he needs to gratify, his senses where his soul does not follow them. A youth really falls in love with another man's kept woman (as in *The Harp of Life*). His conscious and unconscious passion are both directed toward her and carry with them the affection too. Here the only impediment to a complete union is the woman's disintegration, if she be actually erotically disintegrated. It is possible that, in spite of her former liaison, she may become integrated by the youth so that she may be able to be fixed on him, and remain so, unless he should change.

Erotic disintegration is the condition of those

who, with or without insight, feel that they can separate the conscious from the unconscious passion. A man with insight, who feels that he can separate his conscious from his unconscious passion may have insight into the erotic significance of his unconscious acts, but cannot have full insight into the totality of their social relations. In gratifying his senses of touch and his organic senses upon the body of a woman who is unable by her social status and her intellectual attainments, or by her otherwise uncouth or disagreeable qualities to enlist his conscious passion, which is determined not alone by the possession of the usual number of arms, legs, lips, eyes, etc., but by a peculiar quality of each of these members, not to mention mental traits, he is dividing himself against himself, and will remain divided, until the conscious life can assimilate the unsympathetic elements in her make-up. If the fascination is only unconscious, the relation of the man with the loose woman will be marked by much conflict, deep pangs of conscience, and by a strongly impulsive character. On the other hand fascination may in rare cases be only conscious, and may occur on the basis of an unconscious fixation upon a mother imago, in which case a union of this man and any woman will involve only the conscious passion on the part of the man, no matter how much her con-

scious and unconscious passion may be directed
to him. Here is a picture of an unhappy marriage. The wife may be devoted body and soul
to the husband, but he can respond with his
soul only.

J. *Soul and Body Mate*

Erotic disintegration leads to psychic disintegration. It leads to a form of double personality which is somewhat different from the
multiple personality described by psychologists.
But it stands to reason that when there is a split
such as I have mentioned above, between a man's
or a woman's unconscious passion and his or her
conscious passion, and when these two amounts
of desire are directed to two different people,
there is a vital separation in the psyche of the
man or woman itself. We have here a new view
of the eternal triangle in which a man "loves"
two women, sometimes called the soul mate and
the body mate. True love implies the existence
of both in the same woman. When therefore a
woman finds herself regarded as only a body
mate, she can respond only with her body; but
her own soul, if she have one (and we have no
right to suppose she has none), is attracted
toward some other man. She then becomes as
much split as is the man, part of whose personality she shares. And if the other woman

finds herself solely the soul mate of the man thus divided, she is either irresistibly impelled by her unconscious desires to seek the physical love of some other man, so that we have here really five people concerned and not two as there ought to be. We have A, the man, and B and C, his two mates (so called) and D and E, their two adjuncts who supplement for B and C, what they lack in A.

But if, as is sometimes the case, the so-called " soul mate " of A is a woman whose passions are not enlisted, but only her affection, who has, in other words, repressed her passions, we have a woman who is no woman, or is only half human, and no part woman, the other part being virtually sexless. Such a human, ostensibly woman, but not really woman on account of repressed passion, is one whose health, and consequently all her performances are far from being complete and wholesome, on the principle that no human female can really be a woman who is not or who has not been a mother.

Let us also consider the triangle from the point of view of the woman with two mates, a body mate and a soul mate. We find a certain difficulty in imagining this. For the woman who is the apex of this pentagram is very unlikely to have the two kinds of mate. For the woman whose " body mate " does not succeed in being her soul mate is much rarer than the man who is so unfortunate, because men are better educated and have more insight as a general rule than women. A woman whose marriage is unsuccessful on account of repressed passion (and there are almost no women without passion, either expressed or repressed) generally, on account of the repression, lets it express itself as it will in indirect forms, and lives on with her husband in externally placid married relation. She is, by hypothesis, one whose husband is her soul mate alone, and not her body mate. Therefore she will have her affections enlisted, and, as the two are thus partially sympathetic, they let it go at that. They may or may not have children. If they do, their children will miss something from their home life, they know not what. Either it will be the father's occasional caress of the mother, or vice versa, or some of those apparently trivial tender acts that create in the home the atmosphere of perfect love. The children will go forth into the world deficient in the proper foundation of love emotion, partly at least from having been strangers to it in their childhood's home.

K. *Sympathy*

True sympathy cannot exist between husband and wife so defectively married. For sympathy means an identity of feeling, or a tolerance on the part of one of the pair, for the emotions felt by the other. Now in cases where the wife's unconscious passion is not directed toward the husband, the emotions associated with that unconscious passion cannot, in the nature of love itself, be tolerated by the husband. No husband that is himself an erotic unity can tolerate the conscious or unconscious passion of his wife being directed to any other person than himself. With such a wife he cannot have true sympathy. And, *mutatis mutandis* the same may be said of the wife whose husband's conscious passion is directed to her, but his unconscious passion is deflected from her, either fixated upon the husband's mother imago or attracted outside of marital bonds by some other woman.

Therefore in view of the thousand ways in which a marriage may be at least a partial failure, it is of the most vital importance to secure the conditions in the up-bringing of boy or girl where there may be the deepest insight into the nature and divisibility of passion. Let it never be overlooked that "love" as ordinarily understood, means both affection and passion, and that passion is in most people, in all people without insight, both conscious and unconscious at the same time. Conscious passion is what the man and woman are willing to admit to themselves; unconscious passion is what most people either do not know they possess, or from which they feign emancipation. Conscious passion is expressed in the ordinary endearments, caresses and acts of love of all kinds; unconscious passion is expressed, unknown to the individual, in almost all of his or her actions, which are generally attributed, however, to quite other causes.

Love sympathy between married people can exist only when some or all of the unconscious, as well as the conscious, passion is directed by the wife to the husband and, at the same time, by the husband to the wife. Most normal marriages begin that way, and the gradual decrease of the love sympathy is observable under conditions that become less favourable to it externally, such as sickness, loss of money or other economic pressure. Without insight there is hardly any help for this loss of sympathy. But with insight there is the greatest probability that from the beginning each will have seen, and will continue to see, the other as they really are; and, having seen each other as they really are, they will have taken each other as they really are, and not with any erroneous preconceptions due to lack of insight. And having taken each other as they really are, they will not be disappointed in each other, and thus have a fancied cause for mutual resentment and recriminations.

L. *Lack of Insight in the Bride*

Due to lack of insight the majority of young women enter matrimony without knowledge of what may be required of them quite contrary to their expectations, and most men marry with a very strong bias toward requiring of their wives certain duties and spiritual attitudes that they think need not be discussed before marriage. So they not only do not consciously know their fiancées, but through lack of insight many a man has no means of finding out previous to marriage whether or not the woman he thinks he wants to marry has directed, or is even able to direct toward him her unconscious passion.

For it is an unfortunate fact that many women, particularly in modern civilized society, are unable to swing their unconscious passion over to their husbands, because of an early fixation on the father imago. In addition to this many a girl on her wedding night is treated to an unexpected impetuousness on the part of her husband, which repels permanently her unconscious passion for him, even though it might have been directed to him before. Consciously these young women, of both classes, may continue to feel passion toward their husbands, but the unconscious passion is, in the second class,

driven by the apparent brutality back to infantile channels of gratification and, no matter how
well the husband may behave later, the wife, just
because her passion is and remains unconscious,
will be unable to control it, and surrender it to
the very man of all men to whom she consciously
most desires to give up all of herself.

M. *Insight Necessary for the Groom*

It is in the power of the husband in the early
married life, if he himself has insight, so to behave himself toward his young wife, that she
will get insight for herself. No amount of verbal
instruction on his part will avail to accomplish
what a moderate amount of reserve and control
on his part will surely effect. For so surely as
he abandons himself to the gratification on her
body of his own conscious and unconscious passion, will she inevitably and unconsciously, and
absolutely rationally, regard him as uncontrolled, and therefore as a spiritual infant and
not an adult. She will be driven to defend herself against him by the same means as are used
in managing a child,—distraction, diversion, in-
direction, wheedling, beguiling and a powerful
appeal to his pity. Unconsciously she will develop certain infirmities, such as colds, headaches,
gastric and enteric troubles, which are in many

instances merely an unconscious defence mechanism devised by the lower levels of her psyche for the specific purpose of preventing him from getting his essentially purely infantile satisfaction of her. Instead of this defence against him she ought by rights not only to feel any need for defending herself, but she ought to wish, both consciously and unconsciously, to make a complete surrender of herself to him, physically and psychically. But one cannot surrender oneself to a child. To do so could not seem other than absolute folly, and least of all will a woman be able to make this surrender of her unconscious passion, if she have no insight. With insight she might be able to reason the thing out to her own satisfaction, that her just born husband is an infant spiritually, but that, with proper training, he might be made into a man capable of true mutual marriage.

I have spoken in the preceding paragraph of the young wife's need of defending herself against the puerile impetuosity and haste of her husband. This need will be the more readily understood by the reader in realizing not only that the actions of this young husband constitute a "total situation," and mark him unmistakably as a child expecting the unstinted and spontaneous caresses of a mother, but also that the total situation, featuring him as a child, contains the factors necessarily determining her actions toward him as essentially incestuous. There is not only the abnormality of a full-grown woman cohabiting with a prepubertal child not her own, but there is also the necessary implication that, if she cannot feel toward him as an adult woman should feel toward her exogamic husband, she must feel toward him as she would feel toward her own son, if she had one, and as she feels toward her own father.

Against this intrafamilial relation Nature herself has set so strong a barrier that unconscious passion itself cannot break it down. In all cases except where there is unusual degree of insight, the total situation is perceived only by the unconscious. So, wherever the total situation in married life contains these elements which constitute the man's puerility, that is, his impetuosity and lack of self-control, the outlines of incest are inevitably present in the picture, and the woman is absolutely unable to control her unconscious passion, no matter how perfectly the conscious passion is directed to her husband. For Nature herself has inexorable laws against inbreeding, and any psychical total situation in married life, in which the man figures as a child, will be perceived by the wife's unconscious as a situation in which she is married to her own son, for only to her own son, and never to another woman's, would she be expected to act as the lack of control of her husband would evidently seem to require her to act.

This is not to say that after a complete surrender on her part, the man is required to exercise control of his unconscious passion. This control is necessary only so long as the wife's surrender is not complete, and control is the only means possible by which to secure such surrender. After the entire amount of woman's unconscious passion is all won over, exultation on the man's part is peculiarly appropriate, and is joined by that of the woman, the two making a perfect harmony. No act, even of violence, will then be misconceived by either. But the fatal mistake is made in many marriages of the man's showing his exultation, of his blowing off steam to the full, so to speak, of opening wide the throttle and speeding up the car before the woman has entered it. Figuratively speaking, the woman in the matrimonial roadster must be given time in which to sit down comfortably, wrap herself well, dispose of necessary baggage and prepare her mind for the trip. But a large number of young husbands are speed fiends and make a quick get-away themselves, while the wife still has her foot on the running-board.

There are men who are unable to control themselves in such a way as not to be speed fiends.

Those are the men for whom woman means only mother. And from them Nature has taken away the possibility of true happiness in married life, by depriving them of ever being able properly to know a woman. For they have not in their mental make-up the intellectual organs wherewith they may perceive a true woman, even where she really exists. Like the babies blinded at birth by the diseases of their parents, such men are, by ignorance of their mothers and fathers, deprived of the proper psychical constitution by means of which to see and appreciate true non-maternal femininity. It has a quality different from maternal femininity.

For such men, on account of their defective mentality, women fall into two classes, mothers and prostitutes; and the irony of the situation is that they make prostitutes of their mothers by making mothers of prostitutes, as is explained in another section. To their wives they transfer their conscious passion for a while, and to the prostitutes their unconscious passion. These two classes contain for them all the women of their world, a world which does not include the women for whom they might feel not only affection but also both conscious and unconscious passion.

But for men normally constituted and brought up, the world contains two classes of women, the mother, who has been successfully outgrown, and a wife. To the former is directed only affection and to the latter passion of both kinds. For these men, the prostitute type of women does not exist, because their social status, their coarseness, their actual mental defectiveness preclude their attracting the conscious passion of the man. Therefore the attraction of only his unconscious passion does not, in such a man, help split his soul as with an ax. For these men a complete transfer of both conscious and unconscious passion has been made, and can be made, to one woman, who, possessing it all, does not have to, and does not want to, share it with any other woman or women.

And the man who seeks, with one set of women, the gratification of the desires springing from his unconscious passion, while he is trying to keep alive a conscious passion for one other woman, is a man with a defectively working psyche, which is about as safe and sane a thing as a broken-backed steamer in mid-ocean with the water pouring into the huge cleft amidships. And the resort to the lower social level for companionship as surely marks the sub-normal man, as does the practice of prostitution almost invariably mark the sub-normal woman. Everybody knows that prostitution is not right, but few know exactly what is wrong with it. Most men, if frankly giving expression to their views upon this question, will say that of course it is wrong, an economic loss and a cause of the rapid spread of venereal disease, and all the other diseases that follow in the wake of that pirate craft, but, with the infantile attitude of helplessness before something too great for their powers of adaptation, they say that human nature cannot be changed, and that, because no efforts to check or prevent the social evil have been successful, they never will be successful. Those with the infantile attitude toward this great problem have never had it brought to their full consciousness exactly what this split in their mental life really looks like from the inside. They say human nature has never changed and cannot be changed.

N. *Does Human Nature Change?*

This may or may not be the case, but, from one point of view, does not enter into the problem at all. Human nature is probably on the average quite as monogamic as is animal nature which, in many of the higher forms, shows the adumbration of true human single-matedness. It is only in the last ten years that scientific thought has presented a suggestion for the solution of the problems of human passion—a suggestion which is tentatively followed in this volume. If one hears that human nature cannot be changed, it is perhaps quite as well if it cannot, for the attempts to change it have been perverted human attempts, and, with all the abnormality in the world, these attempts have failed. Human nature, as seen from the modern analytical point of view, which is the one taken here, is wholesome and progressive. The passions of the sexes for each other are not experienced in their perfection of fullest intensity except by those who are, in every cellular element of their mind-body combination, fused one with another, outlining in large, in their physical as well as their psychical union, the prototype of the creation of a cell from the union of two other cells,—the mode of reproduction characteristic of all higher animal life.

The suggestion of modern analytical psychology toward the solution of the problem of full physical and psychical development for every individual is the theory of the organic unity of mind and body, and the corresponding essential complicity of the unconscious passion with the conscious. This shows, in the clearest and most striking relief, what is actually the total mental and physical situation of the persons whose love is either atrophied from disuse or "misgraffed in respect of years," or disordered in any way whatsoever. No infectious disease has been successfully combated until the specific germ producing it was discovered. No maladjustment of any part of any organism can be reduced or ameliorated, until the exact conditions causing it, have been accurately surveyed and collated. If the course of true love never has run smooth, that is no sufficient reason why it should not some day do so.

Putting into ordinary language the statement about the organic unity of mind and body is more than merely repeating the trite dictum that love should be perfect and each lover should be all in all to the other. This theory definitely points out just what relations in human social life make for retardation in emotional develop-ment, which should not stop or be arrested until it is consummated in the supreme emotion of the loves of a man and a woman for each other. It puts its finger exactly on the spot where the sun-light of scientific truth should be allowed to asepticize the tissues of the social organism. It is with this in mind that I have presumed to in-terest the reader in the complicated permuta-tions and combinations of conscious and uncon-scious passion, and the insight that renders visible the more archaic strata of the emotions of individuals who are human in the fullest sense.

If the innocently erring men and women, in-evitably following the promptings of their uncon-scious passions, can have it brought clearly into their full consciousness exactly what the split in their mental life, caused by their errant loves really looks like from the inside, they will bend all their conscious energies toward knitting together the fracture in their psychic framework, which, though caused by no fault of their own, but by the ignorance of their parents, is nevertheless their own misfortune. And they will realize that, if they are not above forty-five and, in some instances, fifty years of age, they will be able to repair a break in their natures which, if not repaired, leads not only to locomotor ataxia, through the venereal diseases acquired, but also to dementia, melancholia and paranoia. All these are mental disorders of isolation, that is, disorders where the psyche suffers from the result of the individual's separating himself farther and farther from the norms of steadily progressing society. In a sense prostitution is " old stuff," is antiquated morality, is antique social furniture, tattered and riddled with wormholes of . infection, which no modern spirit would tolerate even in a scrap heap, but would burn up for kindlings to start the greater fires of modern social productiveness.

A woman with real insight is not likely to be attracted toward a man with an unconscious passion fixated on his mother imago, because the indications of his attitude toward the other sex, and his ideas of what a wife should be, if not expressed by what he says or does not say, before marriage, are, so to speak, written all over his face and hands, and are visible in his actions; and she naturally steers clear of such men.

But in the case of a woman without insight, without this ability to read the love message in actions that speak far louder than words, in the case of a woman without insight and a man possessing complete insight, we have a woman who is totally at the mercy of the man, when once she is married to him, and who must endure him or flee from him, after she has found out what he really is. Some of the most beautiful marriages result from just this combination, if the man has both insight and real kindness of heart. But if, as is also sometimes the case, he has complete insight and the ideals of an animal, his woman will never be able to be his true wife, for he will alienate her unconscious passion on the wedding trip, and will have to be, as such men are frequently, to be sure, contented with only a fragmentary wife.

O. *Progress in Insight*

Progress in insight on the part of both lovers is shown in the character development of the novel. For example in *Scandal,* Pelham Franklin is represented at first as quite indifferent to Beatrix Vanderdyke, is enraged at her for the trick she has played on him, when, in order to save her name, she makes him gallantly say that he has married her, and finally during the yachting trip, where he tries to punish her, and outwits her into staying with him alone, his conscious and unconscious passion are directed to her. Her conscious passion is won only at the finale.

The same development is shown in the character of Beatrix, who at first is unconsciously attracted to Sutherland York, and next to Pelham Franklin, whom she catches in the nick of time to prevent her name being soiled. Her progress is shown running from the utter absence of conscious passion at the beginning to the sudden and complete surrender at the end. Her insight came like a sunburst, and after it she could see that her selection of him had been completely unconscious, but nevertheless absolutely whole from the first, in spite of the treatment he gave her both at her home and on his yacht.

The girl with insight is aware of the social significance of her feelings. The girl without is not aware of this significance but is absorbed in the feelings themselves, and in the acts which instinctively and unconsciously express them.

With insight the girl knows that the man she is with may, under favourable circumstances, be the father of her children and of her parents' grandchildren. Without insight the girl is attending only to the face and form of the man who is talking to her, playing tennis with her, or dancing with her, and is conscious only of an inexplicable attraction which, on merely conscious grounds, may be even repulsive to her. To a girl without insight, sitting on the ocean beach on an August afternoon, the bathing master, with his brown arms and legs, appeals by his strength to the unconscious passion, which really desires to be overpowered. But her conscious knowledge of his inferior social position and the sound of his uncultivated words overcome these promptings, and, after the interruption to her reading, caused by his passing within her sight, she goes on with her book. He attracted her physically, or she would not have looked at him once. But, her glance having been unconsciously attracted toward him, she sees in him the qualities which will repel her conscious mind.

The unconscious impressions made by one sex upon the other are constantly being balanced by the conscious impressions. If the unconscious impression creates an attraction, as it generally does, in healthy young people of every grade of society, there is an immediate response in thought or action. Either thought or action is then instantly reacted to by an unconscious thought or action, always, and sometimes by a conscious thought or action. A quick glance or a stare, according to the refinement of the individual, whether man or woman, a blush, an accelerated respiration, a lifting of the hand or an inflection of the body or any one of the multitudinous physical or mental reactions of the complicated human organism, may or may not be consciously perceived by either of them.

P. *Sexual Knowledge Not Insight*

Finally one should not make the mistake of supposing that because people have theoretical knowledge or practical experience of sexual matters, they necessarily have insight. Sexual enlightenment only prepares the way for insight, but does not complete it or even assure its being attained. There are many more people with some kind of sexual knowledge or experience than people with insight. Prostitutes and their patrons lack insight. All those who unite in sexual relations not approved by society lack insight to a certain degree. Insight therefore has degrees, from the lowest, in which a couple of children of the tenements have sexual relations with each other, without knowing what may be any of the results or effects of their acts, to the highest, in which a couple with perfect insight take complete control of their love instinct and relate it socially to their entire lives.

But while insight is not necessarily secured by sexual enlightenment, it is impossible without sexual enlightenment, and I use the term here to mean knowledge, theoretical or practical not only of the physiology of sex but also its psychology. For the physiology alone will offer no help, or at most a very little, to the attainment of insight, which is, on the other hand, dependent most of all upon a practical knowledge of the psychology of sex. This in turn is explained most completely by the concept of unconscious passion and its various modes of expression and attachment.

Thus we see that not only is insight not the necessary result of sexual enlightenment, but it is also not possible to communicate it to others by means of ordinary educational procedure. Therefore the indirect methods of sexual enlightenment are recommended for use in schools, the teachers being advised to show the implications in every subject.

In the home the child should be given direct and plainly worded answers to all his questions about himself, his birth and his conception, to the end that the real mystery shall be placed back where it belongs—the miracle of the origin of any and all life. He will then have more insight, or at least be in a better position to get it for himself, than if he were allowed to get his information about the vital relation between himself and his parents from the contaminated sources of servants and companions. From whom should the real information about parenthood come, if not from the parents themselves? Any stories picked up in the street will be regarded by the child with incredulity and with bewilderment, if his parents, the very persons whom those stories most concern, are mute on the subject, or tell him that he has no right to correct information.

A complete insight will enable either one of a mated pair to understand the other fully, to make due allowances for the actions of the other, even to admire a positiveness of spirit involving differences of opinion between them, and finally to love the other for differences of character, instead of transforming all the differences into causes for suspicion and hatred. Suspicion will, through insight, be seen to be a projection of a feeling of guilt upon another person, and hate will be recognized as an all-absorbing interest in the person hated, an interest which is in a sense polluted at its source which is the unconscious mental activity of the hater. Then, in order to understand this purely subjective nature and causation of hatred it will be necessary only to adopt a more adult, and therefore more social, point of view of the actions of the hated person.

A complete insight will enable one to understand clearly a great many preposterous and inconsistent actions on the part of other men and women. When, for example, it is recognized that almost all of human activity is the expression of its unconscious passion, and of the psychical elements out of which the unconscious passion is developed, there will be far more tolerance for the shortcomings of others, and far more ability on the part of those interested, as all with true insight must be, to remedy the defects of our present wofully defective civilization.

Not Hermia but Helena I love:
Who will not change a raven for a dove?
The will of man is by his reason sway'd
And reason says you are the worthier maid.
Things growing are not ripe until their season:
So I, being young, till now ripe not to reason;
And touching now the point of human skill,
Reason becomes the marshal to my will
And leads me to your eyes, where I o'erlook
Love's stories written in Love's richest book.
Midsummer Night's Dream, II, 2, 113.

CHAPTER V

A. *Unconscious Transfer*

THE unconscious passion usually takes a short time to be transferred compared to the time needed for the transfer of conscious passion. "Whoever lov'd that lov'd not at first sight?" is spoken of Leander in Marlowe's poem *Hero and Leander*. The whole context is so characteristic of the traditional attitude of man to woman since the time of Ovid, that I will quote these lines:

" Stone still he stood and evermore he gaz'd
    Till with the fire that from his countenance blaz'd
    Relenting Hero's gentle heart was strook:
    Such force and virtue hath an amorous look.
    It lies not in our power to love or hate
    For will in us is overrul'd by fate.
    When two are stript long ere the course begin
    We wish that one should lose, the other win;
    And one especially do we affect
    Of two gold ingots, like in each respect:
    The reason no man knows; let it suffice,
    What we behold is censur'd by our eyes.

142

Where both deliberate, the love is slight.
Who ever lov'd that lov'd not at first sight?''
Hero and Leander: Sestiad I: lines 163-176.*

But passion will be stirred more quickly and to deeper levels of the unconscious in some persons than in others, according to their erotic needs and the appeal of the object, and is communicated more gradually to the upper level of consciousness. So that the truth expressed in Marlowe's lines must be re-worded so as to say that unless unconscious passion is aroused, as, if it is free, it will inevitably be by the mere presence of an attractive member of the other sex, there will be no true love. But if the unconscious passion is fixated upon the parent imago, it will not be free, and one will not love any one except the parent at first sight, nor at any other time, for that matter, just because love is the

* "It lies not in our power to love or hate" means simply our conscious power. But in our unconscious power, which is so much greater than the conscious, not only lies the power to love and to hate, but also lies the necessity either to love or to hate a person wholly, or, if the psyche be more sensitive to finer influences and therefore more discriminative and analytical, to love and hate the same person at the same time—to love some qualities of the other personality and hate others, both being simultaneously perceptible to the unconscious mentality, and both working independently of each other with the result of drawing the finer fibred individual in two directions.

The unconscious mental activity or estimation is recognized by Marlowe in the illustration of the runners stript for their course, and the innate preference shown for one of two visually similar material objects. The unconscious estimate of quantities is also hinted at in the two ingots.

transfer of both unconscious and conscious passion.

In the *Midsummer Night's Dream*, Shakespeare represents Lysander as making a dramatically rapid transfer of conscious passion from Hermia to Helena, under the power of the magic drops which Puck has squeezed into his eyes. The rapidity of this transfer of conscious passion is an element of the humour of the situation.

It is interesting to note too that Lysander's unconscious passion is evidently intended by the poet to remain throughout fixed upon Hermia, his first love, a circumstance that causes his elaborate defence of his action in laying the fancied change of heart to reason. He even goes to the extent of openly saying how much he hates Hermia, which is another indication of the steadfastness of his unconscious passion for her.

These transfers of conscious and unconscious passion, however, are later ones, accomplished by people whose unconscious passion has been free, and is made from one adult love to another. It is somewhat different in the average case where the transfer of conscious passion is made upon a basis of an unconscious passion that has been freed from the parent imago and has been in a state of latency, and now is transferred permanently to a life mate. We pass therefore next to a consideration of the transfer of conscious passion of the average person.

B. *The Transfer of Conscious Passion*

The conscious passion of the child, in so far as it is developed, and similarly its unconscious passion, is directed toward the parents and brothers and sisters. At first it is strictly intra-familial. But if there is no family, it may or may not, as in orphan asylums, be developed at all. A picture of a girl in such a situation developing it spontaneously, has been given in *Daddy Long Legs,* by Jean Webster. It might be more clearly stated by saying that the child is naturally a clinging vine, and will cling to any person, with whom it is thrown into close relationship, if that person shows it affection. And, in the child, affection, which is conscious, is shown for the people who do it favours, and passion, or, at any rate, those separately existing elements out of which later organized adult passion is composed, is unconsciously felt for the same persons. This unconscious passion is manifested in the desire to kiss and be kissed, to fondle and be fondled, to be cuddled, to romp with and to "stick to" the person or persons, constituting the immediate family. Sometimes the most loved person is the mother, sometimes the father, sometimes a relative who takes the place of a missing mother, sometimes even a servant.

C. *The Reactions of the Boy*

A boy who has, and is much in the company of, a mother who is young, beautiful and altogether charming, shows his humanity at a very early age by falling in love with his mother. At the earliest age she is quite as much all in all to him as is a young wife to a husband. She is more, for she fills all his conscious as well as his unconscious needs, both nutritive and passional.

At a later date he sees more of other people, and takes most satisfaction in the company of, and in contact with, those people who most nearly fulfil the requirements which the mother fulfilled. He sees one girl with a pretty face, one with beautiful hair, one with wonderful eyes, all of which his mother had for him, another with a physical form which later will coincide with the specifications made by his own growing nature. Later still, at the age of puberty, the boy will be unconsciously aroused by any, or all of the characteristics of one and another girl.

In the meantime, his actual mother has been growing older. Not infrequently she is drawn away from him by the new attractions of other babies of her own. But, if she has no others, she herself will, with truly infantile tendency, stick to him and will help to keep him fastened to her. It is a question whether or not there are boys innately so constituted that they cannot be drawn away from the "mother person" to any other woman. There are surely cases where a boy is apparently unable to give up his mother attitude, but there is no proof that a change of environment, which in these cases rarely occurs, would not enable him to transfer his passion.

The transfer of the passion to another woman than the mother person (mother, sister, aunt, etc.), is necessary for the subsequent welfare of the young man. The time at which this takes place is ordinarily around the time of puberty, but both the time and the rapidity of the transfer differ widely in different cases. Too great a devotion to the boy, on the part of the mother, will retard this transfer and, if the postponement of it is very great, it will never be accomplished.

There is a class of men who marry from their mothers' homes and shift insensibly from the tutelage of the mother, to that of the wife. Frequently they marry so as to have a home; and a home for them means the continuation of the same or a similar home, in which they are the favourite children. This arrangement of the young man's life is frequently the cause of much marital unhappiness in his own wedded life. It is evident that a period of homelessness and hardship is a prerequisite for a happy married life, at least for some men, as only through his being deprived of home influences can such a man take a normal part in a home of his own. For in the home in which he is supposed to be the head he can never be a favoured child, and from his own wife he cannot normally expect the treatment of a mother. No woman can treat her husband as his mother treated him when he was a child, without unconsciously assuming toward him the attitude of a mother toward her own child. The attitude of a mother toward her child, in so far as it affects the unconscious passion of the mother, is complicated with the incest barrier, and, just because of this barrier, no wife who is trained by her husband to regard him as a child can transfer to him her unconscious passion, which is an essential part of the relation between husband and wife.

And from the man's point of view, too, if, because of shifting immediately from one home (his mother's) to another home (his wife's, not his wife's *and* his), he has been trained by his environment to look upon all home women as mothers, he, too, will be unable, because of the incest barrier, to transfer to his wife his unconscious passion, a transfer which is an essential part of the relation of the husband to the wife. Both the transfer of the husband's unconscious passion to the wife, and that of the wife's unconscious passion to the husband are necessary to a complete and perfect union. Without either of these, the relations between the two are defective, either where the wife's unconscious passion is directed to the husband and his is fixated upon his mother imago, or where the husband's unconscious passion is directed to the wife, and hers is fixated upon her father, brother, uncle, cousin, or grandfather imago.

The desirable reaction of the boy, therefore, is a change from being, as it is normally, directed first toward the mother person to being transferred to a woman for whom, because of this transfer alone, he can react with a full unconscious passion.

Almost the same statement can, *mutatis mutandis,* be made about the girl and her spiritual change from girlhood to womanhood, the exception being due to the peculiar nature of the physical substratum of her unconscious passion.

The relation between the failure of the boy, or man, to change from the state of having his unconscious passion directed to the mother, to that of its being free for subsequent transfer to his wife—the relation between this arrest of development in the human male and the social evil, is one that has not been duly emphasized. It is one however that is of the most vital importance, and can only be adequately grasped after a long course of education in social hygiene. In brief, for many, if not most men, the resort to the prostitute is an unconscious attempt to find the mother imago in a woman who has, in some respects, the complaisance and accessibility of the mother as she was known to the man when he was a boy. From another point of view, the prostitute is the mother, with the incest barrier removed, while the wife, from whom the man rebounds, is the mother (with the incest barrier).

D.   *Choice of a Mate*

Whether a man has or has not a conscious ideal according to which he chooses a life mate for himself, he has yet an unconscious pattern. A woman's correspondence with this pattern can never be perfect, to be sure, but the more nearly she approaches his unconscious pattern, the more will she attract him unconsciously. Unmistakable indications of this attraction will be clearly manifest to other people, according to their intuition, but probably not to the man himself, who, having no conscious ideals, is dominated only by the unconscious pattern. Various feelings on the part of different women may easily be imagined, if we cause them to reflect on this aspect of their attractiveness.

But for the unfortunate fact that the unconscious pattern in such men *may* be a mother imago, which carries with it the essential infantility of the man, such an unconscious ideal on his part would be the safest foundation on which a woman could build a love relation with such a man. For the unconscious, containing so large a proportion of his mental activities, would gradually become firmly attached to her personality, and her assurance of his fidelity to her would be absolute.

The difference, however, between a man's choice of a woman being dominated by a mother imago, and a choice not so dominated, is an exceedingly important difference, as we have seen that, where the mother imago is the main factor, there is always present in the relation between the man and the woman, the unconscious incest factor, which prevents his transferring to her the entire amount of his unconscious passion. Where there is no dominant mother imago, the unconscious passion may be transferred to the woman without restraint or inhibition.

In the case of the man whose choice is dominated by the mother imago, we might reasonably ask who is making the choice. Is it the man or his mother imago? One would naturally suppose that a woman would rather be chosen by the man himself than by the unconscious mother imago, living in his psyche and, practically dictating his preference for special kinds of women and actions of women. Women here and there, liberated by the modern feminist movement, are beginning to realize this in a sort of unconscious way; but not even so deeply intuitional a thinker as Ellen Key has apparently comprehended the very great importance of the unconscious thought mechanisms.

It would be all well and good if a woman could be assured that the man she was attracting had the proper normal kind of love for her, that she was attracting him because of herself and not because of her resemblance to some one else —his mother. Mr. B. could be presented to Miss C. by one who knew whether Mr. B's psyche had in it a crystallized mother imago, and who could say: "Allow me to present Mr. B., sufficiently adaptable to be attracted by any wholesome young women, and not dominated by a mother imago!" If, after some months of friendship, Mr. B. showed signs of being attracted, Miss C. would know he was all right, and would satisfy her in the matter of fidelity, if he did not in any other respect. If she liked him in other ways, she need have no doubt as to his making her a good husband, and a few months should be enough to clear her mind upon this point.

In most cases of long wavering between accepting or rejecting a man, the woman is usually assailed by doubts caused by her unconscious perception of the faulty action of the man, and frequently in this very matter of the domination of the mother imago. Without deep natural insight, or the penetrativeness given by the analytical psychology, no woman can tell the Dominant-Mother Imago man from the ordinary adaptable man. But it would be exceedingly valuable to her if she could, because she never can be permanently happy with the one, and can be with the other. A careful study of the mental mechanisms involved in the nature and activities of the mother imago will be required before any one can begin to form a reliable estimate of the character of a prospective mate. The more complicated society becomes, the more difficult is this detection of unconscious traits. In times when the male was chosen by the female after a fight between several males to see who was the stronger, the better man was quite evident. But at the present time, when so many of the factors determining future conduct are repressed by society into the unconscious of the individual, the best man is not known by his most obvious deeds alone, but by the apparently trivial and irrelevant manifestations of his unconscious trends.

So that, in considering the matter of choice of a mate, we have seen that any preference shown by a man for a certain woman, *may* be due to the presence of the mother imago in the man's psyche, and, if so, he will be able to become a desirable husband only after he has had the imago trained out of him, or dissolved by analytical psychology, or after some radical change in his environment that has naturally caused a completely new viewpoint on his part, with regard to most of the conditions constituting a marriage.

So who makes the choice? When the man thinks he is making the choice, he is being directed, not solely, but almost exclusively, by his unconscious. When the woman begins to think that she is being favoured by his preference, let her carefully examine the total situation, including the overt manifestations of the unconscious of her professed admirer, and make up her mind whether or not she is being wooed by a man who can see her only through an unalterable mother-imago screen. If she is quite sure that there is no such impediment, she may rest content to let the unconscious do its work in peace. But if she feels indefinitely, and thereafter knows from conscious self-examination, that there is something not quite explicable in the actions of the man, she must, in order to be happy herself, either have the man examined by some one who is conversant with such things, or have herself examined. For it is quite as possible that she may herself be the unfortunate victim of an imago ignorantly, and innocently fastened upon her by her father, or some male relative.

When we come to the matter of the woman's choosing the man, we are on similar, if not identical, ground. Bernard Shaw said that the woman always does the choosing and that the man has no part in it whatever. Setting aside for the moment the probability, estimated at about 50%, that the woman herself has a father imago that is practically doing all the choosing, we may consider what the choice consists in, on the part of women not so predetermined by the fixity of the specifications of their unconscious passion.

From the modern feminist point of view, there is no rational cause why a woman should not have a voice in the selection of her mate. If choice be restricted to conscious choice, we should find that, in the majority of women, the proportion of conscious to unconscious mental activity was the ordinary one of at most one in ten. Supposing, however, that woman's natural intuition, in which she somewhat excels man, has the result of making more of the total situation conscious, we might estimate her conscious choice, or the conscious factor in her choice, as varying in different individuals from 10% upward. In almost all cases, there will yet remain a very large proportion of the elements constituting the total situation, that do not at all enter her consciousness.

In all cases, therefore, the choice of a mate is determined by unconscious factors. Kissing goes by favour. The unconscious passion of the woman is really the determining factor in any so-called choice of hers. Therefore the only way in which a woman can increase the conscious factor in her largely unconscious choice is by bringing unto consciousness, more of the elements which enter into the balance. I am not for a moment recommending this as a general procedure, advisable for all. But I do wish to emphasize the fact that a choice of a husband which ignores the possibility of his having a fixated mother imago is a very defective choice from the point of view of modern feminism, which is a movement that has as its main feature the bringing into consciousness of much that has been repressed.

" The man's choice of a woman has no meaning, if the man dares not choose at all, or has no prospect of being able to choose something proper." *

* Freud: *Beiträge zur Psychologie des Liebeslebens*, p. 42.

and vice versa, the woman's choice of a man has no meaning, if the woman neither can, nor dares to choose, according to the desires of her unconscious passion.

Serious thought should be given by women to the fact, that in most cases, their bringing up is such that the unconscious component of their passion will be directed only toward those men who do not suggest the persons against whom the incest barrier has been set up by society. Having been brought up always to repress their passion, but particularly in the presence of men of their own social position, they have subjected this passion, which undoubtedly exists in all women, to a pressure that is especially strong in regard to its expression toward equals. Toward inferiors their affection has rendered them rejective, and they naturally give this possibility less conscious thought.

What must be the effect of rendering unconscious a passion that would naïvely be expressed toward men whom their affections would spontaneously make them approve? Repressed in the direction of the father-brother class and blanketed by lack of affection in any other direction, it is no wonder if the entire passion is repressed, both conscious and unconscious. If, then, they are courted by men of their own class, and are, as they will be, prompted to give unconscious expression of their own response, in acts that, in spite of conscious rejection, nevertheless clearly indicate their fundamental approval of such a man, they will surely develop a behaviour that will be most inexplicable to their companions. Always on the verge of a conscious expression of their passion, and yet consciously resisting it all the time, because of the fact that passion has been imprinted with the very stamp of incest, they will shrink from facing the most vital relations between themselves and their suitors, relations which, if allowed to come into consciousness, could be discussed freely, and in regard to which much wholesomeness could be liberated that otherwise would be confined in the unconscious, where it is most likely to become unwholesome, or is liberated only in symbolical or substitute forms, that cause much misunderstanding, because they never are what they seem to be—eccentricities, whimsicalities, caprices, to mention the least malignant, or, in more serious cases, neuroses and psychoses.

E.   *Impediments to Choice*

Before engagement for marriage the man's unconscious passion is either free or fixed. If it is fixed, it is upon the mother imago, and, if free, it may be temporarily attached, now to one prostitute and now to another. If prostitutes are sought by the man with the fixed mother imago, the unconscious passion whose desires he is attempting to satisfy, is impossible completely to gratify. Therefore he never gets complete satisfaction from any one of them. His tension is not completely relaxed even for a moment. There are conflicting elements in the total situation that render impossible his perfect relaxation. In the prostitute this conflicting element is the absence of the qualities of the adorable mother, and their replacement by tone of voice, gesture, odour, and what not that are somewhat repellent. If the object of illicit love has not these discrepancies with the ideal imago formed on the early mother impression, but is charming in all these respects, possibly even more so than the real mother was, she will satisfy the man's lower levels of unconscious desires, and possibly some of the desires of the upper levels. He wants her beautiful, and spirited, well spoken, agreeable and lively, and passionate, all of which are possible with a woman of pleasure. But a woman, to fill all desires arising from conscious, as well as unconscious passion, must be regarded with affection by those whom he regards with affection, admired by those he admires, respected by those whom he respects. By the very fact of his clandestine relation with this woman he prevents the gratification of these desires. In this he is obliged to separate his desires into two groups. In one are those he may gratify in the loose woman's company, in the other those he cannot thus gratify. On the principle that half a loaf is better than no bread, he elects thus to make a partition of his personality, in order to gratify the desires that he thinks he can, and to secure. at least a partial relaxation of his tensions. I should like to be able to say that he consciously makes this separation between parts of himself, but I do not think it would be true, for he does not realize that his conscious desires, springing from his affections, are a part of himself. When he goes to the residence of the detachable or semi-detachable woman, he represses the desires arising from affection. He might as well take off one of his arms or one of his legs, for he cannot put back the one any more than the other.

The affectionate side of his own nature, where it concerns women, is most closely connected with his mother, or with women of his mother's class. In leaving, for the time being, that class and seeking the company of one of a lower class, he is extinguishing that part of his nature. In his relations with the loose woman, unconscious passion for his mother is active in his soul, and determines his choice of her out of other loose women. As the incest barrier is not in this case present, being operative only among women of the mother class, he can get the satisfaction of the desires arising from his unconscious passion without any inhibitions whatever, provided the conscious inhibitions have been rendered unconscious. But in some men this is not possible.

The man finding a woman who filled all his unconscious, and conscious passionate desires, and presented qualities enlisting his own affections too, but not those of his family and friends, or who even alienated all his friends and relatives might remove to another community, and, if all went well, form new social relations under another name, gradually enlarging them until his need for social relations was filled. In case the woman of his choice was congenial to him in every respect and wished to have, and to bring up, children, and herself play a part in the community life, she would then cease to be a loose woman, and would become integrated with the community. After a reasonable time they might even reveal their identity. But this is a rare or even supposititious case. For no woman will become loose in this sense, unless she is seeking, unconsciously, the gratification of desires emanating from an imago that has become fixed in her own psyche. If in her own psyche the unconscious desires were free, they would attach themselves naturally to the first man who possessed her wholly, and they would be wholly transferred to him, and finally and forever. But with a father imago, she is unable to make this attachment and transfer, because the specifications of it are so numerous and so rigid. Therefore she is doomed to fail on her first attempt to secure the relaxations of her own tensions, and similarly to fail on every subsequent attempt. And yet she is driven by the urge of her unconscious passion to continue to attempt, either literally or symbolically, to secure the relaxation above referred to. No wonder if, meeting one new man after another, she will still fail to find in each of them what she has missed in the last of the preceding series.

F. *A Radical Difference*

This indicates a radical difference existing in people, both men and women—difference that must be based on deeply unconscious tendencies —the difference namely between the people who need much, and those who need little variety in their lives. Those who need much variety are the ones who will probably be inconstant in love, and, in view of the researches of modern analytical psychology, it is clear what the true unconscious cause of this is.

The relaxation of tensions, which constitutes gratifications of desires, is secured in all people either by a feeling of fitness, of being truly centred, of fulness of some glands or of complete discharge of contents of others, of gentle contrectation, or of a mild or vigorous activity. But, whatever it is, and with whatever condition associated, this feeling is one feeling—the satisfaction feeling. People can be trained, or can train themselves, to gain this feeling in different ways. The satisfactions of childhood are those of skin sensation, muscle activity and of the various erogenous zones. They might be called satisfaction zones. Adult synthetized sexuality differs from infantile, unassembled sexual elements in the inclusiveness of the associational group of those activities which modern life has embraced in love. Every individual has developed one or more satisfaction groups of activities. His main one may be his business, subsidiary ones may be avocations, hobbies or fads of various kinds.

G.   *The Mercurial Character*

Those people who are fickle, mercurial in character, are the ones whose unconscious *imagines* (plural of imago) whether early developed parent *imagines* or late appearing *imagines* of other kinds, are so to speak, crystallized, inelastic and unadaptable. Every new experience is matched up against this unconscious model, and as it is not met by an elastic nature, it is found to be a misfit, and the experience does not satisfy. The satisfying experience does not exist, or, according to the law of probabilities, is not frequent enough to make it possible that in more than one case out of many millions, a man with a fixed imago should meet a woman with a fixed imago, such that each would exactly fit the other. If this were the rule, and not the exception, there would be no conjugal infidelity, because each imago pattern would find another imago pattern fitting it as nicely as the two parts of a torn piece of paper or broken glass.

Why people do not get along well together in married life is because they cannot, and they cannot because either one or the other has a crystallized imago or both have. What causes this crystallization has not been proven. It may be hereditary. It may be acquired. In either case environment or conscious analysis may improve conditions, but no one can tell this till he tries. At any rate, it is worth trying.

The radical difference between people mentioned above, that is, between the mercurial type, who need constant change, and the jovial type, who do not, is the cause of difference of opinion that seem irrational when looked at only from the conscious side, but are evidently quite natural and inevitable, when the unconscious is reckoned in. The person who quickly tires is the mercurial type. He finds no satisfaction in any line of activity and must change and try another.

It would seem that I am here describing a childish trait, that crystallization is a characteristic of old age, and that I am, therefore, misinterpreting situations. But the changeable nature of childhood is in some children due to the superabundant elasticity and ability to adapt, and is a far different thing from the fickleness of the truly mercurial temperament. The adaptable child is willing to accept, and does accept, changing external conditions, but is not too anxious to change of his own accord; the neurotic child with the already crystallized imago is unwilling not to change, craves variety in the insatiable search for external circumstances to fit a fixed condition within him. The adaptable child has no such subjective crystallization calling for specific satisfactions; the neurotic child has. The adaptable child will change, if change be recommended; the unadaptable neurotic child must keep changing external conditions, whether change be socially advisable or not.

The same may be said of the grown up who is not yet adult in the restricted sense. The man must change, whether or not it be advantageous

for him from the point of view of the community.
He is forced by his unconscious crystallizations
to miss true satisfaction in every home, every
business, every place he works, and everything he
tries to do. The *cacoethes movendi* makes the
tramp. And many are the unconscious tramps,
even in high social and business positions. Some
of the most successful business men are unconscious tramps, who have so intensely compensated for their unconscious errancy, that they
have created enormous systems whose keynote is
the expansion of dissatisfaction. Personally,
they never know satisfaction. They do not know
when to stop temporally or where to stop spatially. They never can secure satisfaction, even
from the possession of millions of money, and of
almost unlimited power. Such men are the heads
of big business and they are boils or carbuncles
on the body politic. By their own weight they
crush other individuals into masses of closely
impacted personalities with no room to develop
themselves. The inordinately great and force-
ful men impress their stamp upon the lesser, and
prevent the latter's natural development. Their
opinions, often narrow and erroneous, have an
extravagant authority and dominate society to
its infinite injury. The profit-sharing devices
of some of these men are an acknowledgment of
the error of their way, and the endowment of edu-

cational and research institutions is a sop to the better feeling of the community, but is always kept strictly within narrow spheres of influence. And all this comes of the inability of these men to adapt themselves to their environment, resulting in a gigantic effort to adapt environment to their unconscious, but elaborate specifications, determined by their own inelasticity. The insatiable thirst for power is as much a disease as is the unquenchable thirst for alcohol, or the never to be satisfied craving for drugs, and arises from the same crystallization of the psyche that causes that much more multitudinous evil in common men—prostitution. The magnate prostitutes society to his own personal mental disorder, thereby manifesting infidelity to the best interests of the greatest number of his brothers and sisters.

H. *Psychic Valuations*

Freud * says: " The passionate current that remains active seeks only those women who do not suggest the prohibited incestuous persons. If an impression is received from one person, which might lead to a higher psychic valuation, it works out in arousing not sensuality, but affection, which erotically is unavailable. The love of such men is split in two directions, - which are

* *Beiträge zur psychologie des Liebeslebens,* page 43.

personified in art as the heavenly or earthly
(animal) love.   Where they love, they do not
get sensual pleasure, and where they get sensual
pleasure, they cannot love.   They seek women
whom they do not need to love, in order to hold
off their sensuality from the women they love,
and, according to the laws of ' complex sensitivity ', and ' the return of the repressed ', the
peculiar obstruction seen in psychic impotence
appears, if, in the object chosen for the avoidance of incest, a frequently insignificant looking
trait reminds them of the woman to be avoided."

The " passionate current that remains active "
implies that a part of the passionate current remains passive. *   But it cannot be wholly passive.   It must manifest its activity in some other
form.   Therefore, in the present passage, Freud
is implicitly making a distinction between the
conscious passion, which is equivalent to " the
passionate current that remains active " and the
unconscious passion which is the passionate current that remains inactive.

The active passionate current is conscious passion, and the inactive passionate current is unconscious passion.   The inactive passionate current is not really inactive.   It would be a mistake

---

* *Passion* is derived from the Latin *patior*, to suffer, or to *allow*
or *be acted upon*, so that it seems a contradiction to speak of active
passion.   But the modern view of emotion is different from the
ancient one, and passion is regarded now as a reaction to a love
stimulus—a reaction of sufficient intensity sometimes to enter
consciousness, but not always.

to call it passive. It is repressed into the unconscious, where it is possibly even more active by virtue of its being confined there, and strives in every possible way to express itself symbolically in overt actions, since it cannot express itself literally. According to the similarity feeling or feeling that two sense qualities are similar, a feeling which is itself a sense quality differing from the other two, any activity may take the place of that activity originally desired, provided only that the amount of, or intensity of, the familiarity feeling is great enough, even if it is not absolutely complete. Thus substitute sensations and substitute actions may take the place of the sensations and actions first desired. Complete satisfaction would remove all desire, until the subjective conditions themselves changed, but the partial satisfaction, secured through the substitute, leaves always some satisfaction yet to be gained. This results in a connection being formed between satisfaction and frustration,— every such satisfaction being part frustration. This condition is well illustrated in its extreme form in masochism, where the frustration (pain) becomes apparently an integral part of the pleasure.

I. *Debasement of the Love Object*

Continuing from the place last quoted (p. 167), Freud says: "The chief protective means against such disorder (psychic impotence) that the man avails himself of in this splitting of love, is the psychical debasement of the sexual object, while the normal over-valuation of the sexual object is reserved for the incestuous object, and her surrogates. In proportion as the requirement for debasement is fulfilled, sensuality can fully express itself. . . . Generally, also those in whom the affectionate and the passionate currents have not regularly flowed together, have a love whose development has been arrested. Perverse sexual aims have been retained by them, whose non-attainment is felt as a perceptible loss of pleasure, but whose attainment, evidently, is possible only with debased, under-rated sexual objects."

That is, the woman is debased by the man so that he may be able to gain, from her, infantile satisfaction (familiarity feelings of satisfaction). He debases her by regarding her as less than woman. As less than woman, she can give him satisfactions that a woman could not, because, the true woman has assembled the diverse components of infantile erotism (the pleasures from the stimulations of the different erogenous zones), into the unity of adult love, and the restriction of the love act, on the man's part, to any, or several of these uncombined elements is a cause of displeasure to her, while the man derives his greatest pleasure from the restricted areas, and, having secured his own acme of pleasure, he is unable to act in such a way as to increase the woman's to her maximum, without which he will not satisfy her, nor in the end will she satisfy him.

In the debased love, however, the man has no regard to whether he is satisfying her, being concerned solely in his own state of mind, a condition in which, as before stated, he is merely autoerotic. A man's power to debase a woman is dependent, therefore, on his own infantility. The woman is only debased, and never ennobled, by the infantile man. The infantile man can only debase his woman, and can never ennoble her. That is not to say that the woman is never debased by any other cause than by the infantile man. She may be debased by her own lack of development. The fact that one-third of all prostitutes are below the average intelligence is a proof of this. These are below their proper intelligence age. The other two-thirds are below their proper emotion age, which implies an arrest in the development from unassembled erotic elements toward the fully synthetized adult love instinct that demands totality. This accounts for the debasement of the woman, and explains how she becomes debased. Methods preventive of this debasement have never yet been adopted. Fully to carry them out would require an amount of money spent upon public education that would stagger the present generation of men. Therefore modern society tacitly, assumes that the economic waste of the social evil is a less expense than would be the attempt to develop the individual, both emotionally and intellectually.

Man generically debases woman individually, so that individual men can get a relaxation of a certain kind of tension through regarding women generically as debased. In so doing he either debases himself, or is himself debased, on account of the incomplete development of his love instinct.

The incomplete development of the love instinct has an inevitable effect upon the development of man's intellectual ability, and upon his social, financial and every kind of practical success. Frink * reports a case where a man, a canvasser for a certain advertising medium, became troubled by a doubt that the return that he promised his prospects was not after all what he was leading them to expect. This doubt was,

* *Morbid Fears and Compulsions*, New York, 1918.

upon analysis, revealed to him as a transmutation of a doubt concerning his own love affair. He had deceived a girl under pretence of marriage. His natural doubt about his giving full value in his love life, was unconsciously transmuted into a doubt about his giving full value in his business life, and materially interfered with his success, as it lessened his commissions to a considerable extent. It will be thought by some men that they can be direct in one part of their lives, and indirect in all others, and there may be some men—but there are a few exceptions to every rule.

It may be asserted that physiologically, this man's relation to this girl was perfectly normal. About this, however, there can safely be said to be some doubt, as the physiological love reaction has been shown to be dependent upon the psychic factor. Psychic impotence is only an extreme form of this physical-psychic interrelation. It is not likely that the physiology of love will be perfect, if the mental side of it is defective in any way. In order to gratify the desires arising from his unconscious passion, this man was repressing into the unconscious, some relations of factors in the total situation, which would be necessary not only to a perfect psychical, but also to a perfect physical love. Had his physiological relation with the girl been perfect, he would have had no doubts whatever, about marrying her, and the social relations included in the total situation, would have been satisfactory. He would have been completely inspired to make her his wife, and to face the world with her.

To any one who says that the illicit loves of men for prostitutes are physiologically perfect, I should reply that not only are they not, but cannot be, for the reason that the infantile and autoerotic nature of the love for women of the debased class, makes complete transfer of both conscious and unconscious passion and of affection impossible. If this transfer is made, the love is perfect, and the woman is not debased. But the complete transfer can be made only by the really adult man, adult both intellectually and emotionally.

It should be remembered that in the instance given above, the *connection* between the man's love and business life was perfectly real, but absolutely unconscious. There is quite as likely to be a real connection between the business and the love life of the all average men which, though completely unconscious, is quite as real as if it were consciously sensed. And if the same holds true of women, it is a mistake to employ as teachers of young children, unmarried women, or women not mothers, because the only fit person to handle young children, is a mother. She alone will be able to behave most consistently toward them. The unconscious psychic relation of an unmarried woman teacher to a child is that of an older sister to a younger brother or sister, and the unconscious psychic relation of a child to the unmarried woman teacher is that of the younger member to an older sister, a relation in some cases very beautiful, but in the average, not.

J. *The Familiarity Feeling*

The feeling of satisfaction is one composed largely, if not wholly, of the feeling of familiarity, and, paradoxically, it is the lack of satisfaction (which implies also a lack of familiarity) that accounts for the tedium of the unimaginative people who are bored by what they think is too much sameness. These unimaginative, mercurial people already referred to are, like every one else, searching for satisfaction and are not finding it, because they fail to get that familiarity feeling which comes from a complete correspondence between the subjective form and the objective conditions that are looked for to fit it exactly. As they do not get complete correspondence between their desires and reality, they do not get the familiarity feeling they are striving for. The only sameness in their situation is that of the misfit. Every new experience is the same misfit to their wishes as the last experience was. Therefore are all the uses of this world to them weary, flat, stale and unprofitable. But to the person who has an adaptable psyche, with no parent imago or any other kind, privileged, therefore, to fit into any situation, the correspondence between the ego and the world of reality is perfect, the familiarity feeling complete, the satisfaction perpetually recurrent. One cannot help thinking that this is the normal way for humans to react to their environment.

It is not difficult to imagine why this must be the case, if we picture to ourselves the earliest experiences of life. The infant is put to the breast for its first meal, after sufficient time in which to become reasonably hungry. It feeds until its cravings are satisfied, whereupon it goes to sleep until it is hungry again. At a second feeding, the pangs of hunger are a second time stilled, but this time with the first opportunity for that familiarity feeling of perfect satisfaction,—a feeling which filled its ego after the first mundane meal, and which is now repeated with the additional familiarity feeling of satisfaction. Every subsequent satisfaction is but the replica of that original prototype. It should never be forgotten that the familiarity feeling is a feeling different in quality from the full-stomach or warm-hands-and-feet feeling, and that, while it may be associated with sensations of comfortable fulness of the stomach, it emphatically is *not* those sensations, which are in the gastric region, whereas the familiarity feeling is one that illuminates the total situation.

It may be said that the feeling of distress which is predominant in the infant ego before the first, is also the same as that before the second meal, and that here we should have another familiarity feeling quite as good and definite as that associated with satisfaction. But the fact that the distress is associated with apparently aimless movements of the entire body, while the satisfaction feeling is connected with definite and limited activities in hands and organs of deglutition, should make it clear that the two feelings are very different in the degree of sameness. In other words, the squirming, wriggling, crying and getting red in the face are irradiated activities, whereas those of absorbing the meal are concentrated, giving them a much greater unity and identity. Therefore the familiarity feeling of satisfaction is primarily integrative, whereas the not to be denied familiarity feeling of distress is fundamentally disintegrative.

There can be no doubt that the integrative feeling of familiarity associated with satisfaction is going to play a much greater part in the development of the indivdual than the other, and is going to be the quality that will distinguish the really successful life from the emotional wreck. The mercurial people, the fickle, unreliable, unsteady, unfaithful, shifty, unpersistent, undependable, unemployable people of the world, are those who can never get satisfaction out of anything they do, and the reason why they cannot is that they lack just this pliancy in their own contacts with the world of reality that will allow them to fit into it closely enough to cause a perfect correspondence between their desires and their deserts, and give them the feeling of familiarity, which is satisfaction, and all the health and strength and happiness which a continuance of that feeling carries with it. Fortunate indeed are the people who are innately endowed with so much adaptability that they are disconcerted and misfitted by nothing! This need not mean that they are unduly changeable. For changeableness, as now must be quite clear, is in direct proportion to maladaptation. The misfits have to try another situation. But no matter how gradually or how completely they shift their environment, there is that in their unconscious which will always prevent their finding a perfect correspondence between their desires and their surroundings. The man who is perfectly satisfied is not going to make any. radical change in his life. On the other hand, the man who is continually on the move from one occupation to another, will inevitably be of less economic value than the steady man, as he will use up so much of his energy in the very details of adapting himself each time to his new surroundings, to which he is driven by the unconscious urge from the old ones, where also he spent much time in all too unsuccessful attempts at adjustment.

K. *Identity of Satisfaction*

" The sexual instincts find their first objects according to the values set by the ego instinct, exactly as the first sexual satisfactions were experienced in connection with the functions of the body necessary to the maintenance of life" (Freud, *op. cit.* p. 41).

The experiences producing the satisfaction feeling in the case of gratifying hunger, relaxing fatigue or getting gratification of the desires arising from conscious and unconscious passion, all produce the same satisfaction feeling. It is all one feeling, whether the desire is directed toward pleasures derived mainly from a part of the body or toward purely mental pleasure, so-called. The comfortable sense of fulness, but not overloadedness, of relief from pressure, of dimming of too bright a light, of softening too loud a sound, of replacing noise with musical sound, is all the same sense of gratification that was experienced after the first or second meal of life, and differs only in its extensity, covering now less, and now greater, areas of the personality.

Thus we can get comfort and discomfort at one and the same time. We may have warm hands and cold feet, and vice versa, may sit facing a fire, and have a draft of wind on our back. We may have physical pleasure and mental pain or vice versa. Some elements in the total situation will be pleasant and others unpleasant, and the natural human tendency is to drive the unpleasant ones into the unconscious. The attention naturally focusses on the pleasant elements of the total situation, integrating them, and ignores the other elements, leaving them to integrate themselves as best they may. When we are in a situation containing both pleasant and unpleasant elements, our attention vacillates between them. Now the pleasant elements come into full consciousness, and while the unpleasant ones are there, they are not attended to, for a brief space, during which they become as unconscious as the most unconscious thought. They may be permanently relegated to the unconscious, even though they be actual things making real sensations on actively responding sense organs. Yet they have their existence not in consciousness, but just as much in the unconscious, as if they were last year's forgotten trivialities.

This swinging back and forth of attention from the pleasant elements of the total situation to the unpleasant elements, takes place at different tempi on different occasions. Sometimes attention is given for a greater length of time even by the same person to the pleasant experiences (including thoughts, for thoughts are but subjective experiences) than to the unpleasant ones. Sometimes more time is spent in keeping unpleasant experiences in consciousness than pleasant ones, but there is a reason for this, for the people who do it all the time are gaining pleasure from the bringing of displeasure into consciousness. In an average collection of people some will always be found who have made a habit of dwelling upon the unpleasant things of existence. " Some one is always taking the joy out of life!"

Those who look upon the dark side of life do so because they have found a satisfaction in that kind of activity. Either they have acquired a greater eloquence in expressing their views of the miseries of existence, or they think they elicit sympathy from other people, or in some way they gain the familiarity feeling of satisfaction from each and every situation where the majority of factors are unpleasant, or from subjective situations produced by themselves in which the unpleasant factors are emphasized and magnified.

If we imagine an individual in a situation not too destructive, out of which he can still gain some pleasure from expressing his unfortunate condition in words or actions, he would hardly be human, if he did not take some enjoyment in lamenting his fate. If he must merely lament and feel pain and get no joy of expression at all he will deteriorate in his very tissues.

CHAPTER VI

THE EMOTION AGE

EVERY one has a mental age, measurable by the "intelligence tests", which have been so much elaborated lately. According to them, a man or a woman may have been born in 1880, for example, and now, though forty years old, may be mentally only eight. Similarly with regard to passion every one may be said to have an emotion age, which in some cases differs widely from their mental or intellectual age. The emotion age will be ascertained by observation and experiment upon what people take pleasure in, and it will be found that, just as the capacity for remembering series of numbers, and for other mental performances, increases with the mental age of the individual, so will the emotional reaction differ, and become more complex with his advancing emotion age. The infant age will be dependent upon mother and mother surrogate for most of its pleasures, the childish age on the pleasures derived from its muscle instinct, or will be marked by the predominance of sadism, masochism, exhibitionism, narcissism or the fixation of the unconscious passion upon the parent imago.

At some future time it will be possible to tell a young couple what is their emotion age, and whether or not they are of the same emotion age, and if not, what will be necessary for them to do, in order either to advance to the age of emotional maturity, when it will be proper for them to marry, or for one of them to advance to the emotion age of the other, without which parity of emotion ages it would be folly for them to attempt mating.

For it must be quite evident to the reader that the majority of unsatisfactory marriages, and all the unhappy ones, are unsatisfactory or unhappy because of a disparity of emotion ages between man and woman. Either the man is adult, and the woman a child, or the woman is adult, and the man is a child, psychically, that is emotionally.

A. *The Five Ages of Man*

The different ages of man from the emotional point of view, so far as they are marked off by the development of the unconscious passion, have been tentatively proposed by analysts as somewhat as follows.

The emotional age of infancy is characterized

by complete dependence upon the mother or person acting as mother. Ferenczi * has gone into the divisions of this age, dividing it into the periods: (1) of unconditional omnipotence, (2) of magical-hallucinatory omnipotence, (3) of omnipotence by the help of magic gestures, (4) of magic thoughts and magic words.

Following the emotion age of infancy, comes the first childhood age, from about four to seven years, during which the earlier repressive activities of the social environment are deepened and their work completed. The second childhood age, from seven to the onset of puberty, is characterized by physical growth and muscular development, and by a partial separation of the child from its parents, a separation in thought only, for rarely do children leave home during this age. This age is the time when natural modesty, shame and similar reticence about sexual emotions originate, which are, however, compensated for, by a self-assertiveness, in the boy particularly, and in the girl by a boyish fondness for rough play. From the fact that the sexuality of the infancy and first childhood age is repressed now, this age has been called the latency period. It is in this latency period that the early memories of infancy become so submerged by rapidly accumulating sensory motor experiences, that it

* *Contributions to Psychoanalysis*, Chapter VIII, pages 186-196.

is thereafter practically impossible for the individual to recall these early times and the emotions then prevalent. But there are still men and women of adult physical and mental age, who yet react emotionally, as if they were children in the latency period.

The pubertal age is from twelve to seventeen, the first figure being the average earliest age for girls, and the second the average latest age for boys. During this emotional age, comes the first natural linking of conscious and unconscious passion in those children who spontaneously develop a degree of insight, but they are comparatively rare. The majority of children, during the pubertal age, are in the process of experiencing, for the first time, one or another of the truly adult sexual emotions, but they rarely, or never achieve the full synthesis of the diverse factors out of which true adult passion is assembled. Frequently in the pubertal age, the sexual emotions are merely intensified, but still separate, excitations of erogenous zones, which tend, during this age, to become unified by the inception of the internal secretions, specifically characteristic of the male and the female human.

The fifth, and last emotion age is that of well-rounded adulthood, wherein the fact is made more vividly patent to the individual that sex is largely psychical, and only partly physical.

The unconscious passion is now completely developed, both conscious and unconscious stimuli
producing reactions which are either repressed
or sublimated, and the capacity of the genital
system spreads so as to take up into its unity
all the emotions that can be felt consciously, and
all the reactions that cannot be consciously perceived, and integrating them into a system de-
signed to function as a unit, which shall involve
every atom of the body, and every tendency of
the mind.

It is in this age that the maladjustments in
emotional reaction, which, in some cases, have
originated in the preceding ages, come to their
most extravagant expression, and it is in this
age that irrationality in man or woman is most
missed when it is absent. Now too is the greatest opportunity for the developed insight, and for
the effect to be produced upon the unconscious
passion, an effect caused by the retroactive influence upon it by the conscious life. In the
earlier ages, results can be obtained best by
indirect means working on the unconscious passions, but in the adult emotion age, the best
results are produced by starting from consciousness and working downward.

This age completes the evolution of the emotions. After the forty or fifty years of adulthood, there begins an involution, but the emo-

tions of this age, while they have been characterized in part by analytical psychologists, do not so
much interest us here, as we are concerned only
with the ontogenetic evolution of the emotion of
love.

B. *True Monogamy*

It must be evident by this time, I am sure, that
the truly monogamous marriage requires, in both
the members of the pair, the presence of recipro-
cally directed passions, of both levels, and that
the absence of either passion in either member is
a calamity, not merely of individual importance,
but of social importance, accounting as it does,
for so much of human infidelity. Mrs. Evans *
tells of a young wife, whose husband did not
fulfil her man requirements, according to the
specifications laid down by her experience of her
father. The father was a quiet man who sat by
the fire after dinner, read the paper, and smoked
a cigar, and was orderly and unexcitable. Her
husband was quite the contrary, would handle
her roughly when he greeted her, smoked ciga-
rettes, throwing ashes and stumps everywhere,
and generally put things in disorder. Because
she had learned in her childhood to expect that
kind of action which she saw in her father, she
expected it in her husband and her uncon-

* *Problem of the Nervous Child,"* New York, 1920.

scious had never really been able to adjust itself to the more boisterous manners of the husband.

It might be asked whether this failure on her part to adjust to the different behaviour of her husband was not a defect in her own character or nervous disposition. It certainly was, but it has never yet been proved that such a defect is innate in the individual, and can never be removed. Can the habit of reacting with pleasurable emotions and creative behaviour be put in the place of the habit, such as we see in this young wife, of reacting with unpleasant emotions and inefficient behaviour to her husband? In other words, can the young wife in question be taught properly to react to the part of her environment furnished by her husband? If she cannot, she will be unable to love him fully, to make a full surrender of her personality to him in a complete transference of her unconscious passion.

This brings in the question of whether the complete transference of passion to one object is necessary or even desirable. It involves the essential point of monogamy, whether it is possible for men or women to be unconsciously monogamous, or it is necessary and inevitable that they should in their unconscious passion be actually polygamous.

Being actually monogamous in the unconscious as well as in the conscious life would mean that the unconscious passion is so well trained that it does not feel desire for more than a definite one mate of the opposite sex. By some students it is thought that this is not possible, and that our instinct for reproduction, being a very archaic, and necessarily permanent one, must be less specifically differentiated than any other instinct, and that the unconscious passion must, therefore, normally be quite errant in its nature, and have no capacity for being trained upon one man or woman.

But in the unconscious passion fixated upon the mother or father imago, we have an example of absolute fidelity to a mental impression. It is a fidelity of the unconscious to a definite specific object. If this is the kind of fidelity expected of the monogamous partner, it would seem that in the kind of fidelity which the man unconsciously has for his mother imago, which drives him to seek gratification in one prostitute after another, we have finally found the fidelity which alone would constitute real monogamy, but strangely enough, while it is internally an absolutely undeviating fidelity to one, externally it is the opposite. Convention requires a man to repress his passion for his mother; therefore, such passion is unconscious passion. Convention also requires a man to divert his unconscious passion from his mother or sister to some woman outside of the family. In the man with the unconscious passion fixated upon his mother imago, we see one who is unconsciously monogamous, but consciously, in one sense, polygamous. Of course he does not know that he is polygamous, and from this point of view could not be called consciously so, but there is polygamy somewhere, and it is not in his unconscious, so I shall have to call it conscious polygamy. His polygamous acts are consciously carried out, but they are determined by his unconscious monogamy.

In a man, on the other hand, with no fixation of his unconscious passion upon his mother imago, we have one who may be unconsciously polygamous, but who is or may be consciously quite irreproachably monogamous. Psychically he is able to transfer his passion from his mother imago, to which it is in all men transferred in infancy, to any other woman for whom he feels affection. The man with the fixated mother imago cannot do that.

But the man with the unfixated or free libido, after meeting various women, who appeal to his affection, more or less, but equally to his unconscious passion, finally makes a selection of one of them, and, partly voluntarily, partly involuntarily, depending somewhat upon *her* unconscious reactions, transfers to her permanently the whole of his conscious and unconscious passion. That is to say, more and more his life with her becomes a habit, deeply ingrained into his soul, so that it may be said that he eventually fixates his unconscious passion upon what might be called a wife imago. Such a man then becomes monogamous in every sense of the word. While his affections may go out toward men and women alike, his passion, both conscious and unconscious, is firmly and permanently attached to the personality of one woman. The woman herself may change, but his imago of her once formed and given its lasting outlines in the heat of passion, does not change, so that he may himself even be faithful to a wife who is unfaithful.

C. *Unconscious Bigamy*

True monogamy is only the coincidence of conscious and unconscious passion attached by a man or a woman to one and the same woman or man respectively. If only the conscious passion is attached by the man to the woman, he is not monogamous. He is essentially, because fundamentally and deeply, bigamous, if he marries one woman, while he is unconsciously in love with another—his mother or sister imago. Regarded from this point of view, many legitimate marriages are seen to be virtually unconscious bigamies, for the man is united, in by far the greater part of his ego, to one woman, but in the other (the conscious part) only, is he united to his wife.

It is not inconceivable, either, that a man may be quite monogamous at the beginning of his married life, and afterwards develop bigamous unconscious tendencies. He may succeed in transferring both his conscious and his unconscious passion to his wife, even though he may have had other liaisons of various natures before he married. But, after a year or two of marriage, his wife may change so as to make less appeal to his unconscious passion. If that happens, he is, though perhaps for the first time in his life, a virtual, though unconscious, bigamist. As a matter of fact, if his unconscious passion for his wife grows less, and is gradually transferred to some other woman, he will cease being a bigamist only by getting a divorce from his wife and marrying the other woman. If he does not divorce, but allows the two relations to go on side by side, he is a bigamist according to moral law, if not according to civil law. This is the strongest argument for spreading as widely as possible among all married people, and among those intending to marry, a conscious knowledge of the rôle that is, or will be, played in their marital relations by an unseen force, perceptible only in its effects. It is the strongest possible argument for a conscious study of the unconscious acts that indicate any deviation or deflection of the unconscious passion.

This again raises the question as to whether there be not certain men, whose unconscious passion is not capable of a truly monogamic relation. It may be quite possible that the associative bonds in some people are not strong enough to retain their fidelity to one image. If constancy is dependent upon the direction of the conscious and unconscious passion being the same and directed toward one woman, they may be constitutionally incapable of constancy. It would seem as if constancy is secured only by the conscious mind gaining control over the unconscious passion. This control cannot be secured, either if the individual has not been taught that there is such a thing as unconscious passion, or if the unconscious passion is permanently fixated upon a parent imago.

D. *Good Son, Good Husband?*

There is a popular idea that a good son will make a good husband, the reasoning being that if a man is fond of his mother, he will be more likely to be fond of his wife, that if he stays around home in his youth, he will, after marriage, be likely to spend his evenings with his wife and not neglect her in favour of club meetings or other diversions or relaxations. But the most likely boy to stay around home is one who has formed a strong mother imago in his childhood and, by hanging around his mother during his youth, is unconsciously gaining the satisfaction of the desires which come from that mother imago. This does not mean that the youth will take much conscious enjoyment out of his comparatively domesticated existence. On the contrary he may become ill-tempered, and actually treat his mother shamefully, imposing on her good nature, all the time that his unconscious passion for her is, without his knowledge, forcing him to make demands upon her, with which her own unconscious passion for him drives her to comply, although she does not know why. She slaves to keep him looking well, frequently with no conscious gratitude from him, and responds to his overt abuse of her with conscious bitterness in her own soul, both feelings being overcompensations for their mutual but unconscious passion.

A man may have at the same time both conscious and unconscious passion for his wife, but under circumstances where the wife really represents two persons as objects of the two passions. The object of such a man's conscious passion is the wife as he really sees her, apart from his view of her as a mother imago. But no matter how intense his conscious passion for her may be, he is unable to unite with it his unconscious passion, because it is fixated upon the mother imago. They function for him at different times, or he sees her now as wife and now as mother, but, try as he will, he will never be able to separate from her the mother, and particularly in the most intimate relations of marriage. Along with his conscious passion for her as wife there goes his unconscious passion for her as mother, a passion from which he can never free himself. This is seen in the most ordinary and trivial acts of every-day behaviour. The characteristic of the mother-infant situation which he reproduces with her many times a day, is his need for instant compliance on her part with every demand. Trained by an indulgent mother, he expects his wife to give in to him in every respect, and is impatient if she delays doing for him what favours she is able to do. From his mother he would never learn the art of winning a woman. He has probably won his wife's consent to marry him by an impetuous and sudden onslaught, accompanied by tantrum-like action, which in the infant of adult size is quite effective with some women, as it does indeed represent strength, and strength in man has a powerful appeal to the unconscious passion of woman. She is " set " to go off at this situation. She has yielded to his importunity. He threatens to shoot himself or to run away or to do some other childish thing, if she does not consent to be his wife, and she reacts to that phase which his strength puts on, exactly as the mother has reacted to the child's threat to run away, and to his infant rages.

E. *Child Husbands*

But this is no situation to elicit a woman's unconscious passion for a man, for though it has in it, the one element of strength, it has likewise many components of sheer childishness. If a perfectly wholesome, normal young woman is confronted with a man enacting what is essentially an infantile tantrum in her presence, and concerning her, her perfectly wholesome normal reaction to that situation is to become disgusted with his behaviour, and to tell him to run along and think of something else. She never can wholly admire that course of action on his part, though she cannot say why, and, if she yields to him, it is against her better judgment, which is the unconscious sizing up of the situation as a whole. There is no doubt that she may be a woman on whom such rage on the man's part may have a very potent effect but only in her unconscious passion is it a favourable one to him. It is really more likely to impress her affection, for no woman would want to have any man do himself violence because of her, but would this threat really make her want to marry him?

I have absolutely no doubt that such a man makes upon the unconscious mind of the wholesomely developed woman an unconscious effect of extreme repugnance. If she is unconsciously attracted at all, it is only by the element of strength that he develops in his demonstration of passion. If she could however realize consciously that the strength is mere infantile strength and is devoted to mere infantile aims, she would be certainly repelled. Woman, having in her the germ of future generations, can be appealed to fundamentally only by a situation as widely social as possible. Her arguments to convince herself that she really can love him some time are pure rationalizations. She may indeed think: " If he loves me as much as all this, it will be quite possible for me to come to love him," or: " If I do not marry him, I may make him miserable forever, and I don't want to make any man I like miserable."

If a man has in this manner stormed the feelings of a woman, we may be sure that it is only her surface feelings that have been stirred by the storm. If she yields to the child in him, he is for evermore stamped as a child in her unconscious estimation of him. Her unconscious has not taken him, and never can take him, as a man. He will always be for her a little boy. Her unconscious passion is still unaffected toward him, and remains unaffected, until it responds to the more manly behaviour of another man. And then, married to one man, for whom she cannot experience unconscious passion, she unwittingly falls in love with another, and the way is prepared for tragedy.

From the man's point of view, a marriage like this is prejudicial, not only because she cannot love him with her entire being, but also because he cannot love her, for the reasons I have mentioned above. Forcing her consent by childish means, he necessarily regards her as one whom infantile methods of coercion can, and must, be used in the future. And, regarding her from the angle of a child, he can never see her as other than the only woman visible from the child's angle—the mother. Nor can he see her from the angle of the man with whom she must later really fall in love.

All this is however in the unconscious, for consciously he may form fine adult conceptions of their married life. He may be a successful business man, or with plenty of money power through inheritance, or he may be a brilliant professional man, and yet have the unconscious passion of an infant.

F. *Liberated Unconscious Passion*

On the other hand the man with the completely liberated unconscious passion for the woman he loves consciously will behave quite differently. I say liberated, because the unconscious passion of the man is universally attached to his mother originally and his second birth (that into, the world of adults) consists in his cutting the spiritual cord which binds his unconscious passion to his mother. It is at the time when this cord should be cut, but in some men is not cut, that the actual mother is transformed for him into a mother imago. But in the normal or average man this spiritual separation from both mother and mother imago has taken place, and, for a number of years, all women are alike strangers to him, even his own mother.

Then, when the unconscious passion, which is now equally attracted by all attractive women, is supplemented by a conscious passion for some one woman, with whom he has become more closely acquainted, he is able to transfer to her more and more of his unconscious passion than would have been transferred without the closer acquaintance. The situation begins to involve more and more psychic elements, and every new experience with her is accompanied by pleasure, for the simple reason that he has no preconceived ideas as to how she ought to act. To the man with the liberated unconscious passion, all surprises, and the wholesome woman is full of them, are sources of gratification. Every new light upon her reveals a new beauty. Expecting nothing, because his soul is not full of elaborate specifications made on an old design, he is constantly being treated to an agreeable display of feminine mentality.

With absolute confidence in himself, derived from his lack of multitudinous requirements as to what a woman should be like, he is not nonplussed, confounded and disappointed by any amount of unaccountability in her behaviour. Where the man with the fixated unconscious passion dreads each new revelation, because it *may* not fulfil some diminutive requirement, the other man, with the free unconscious passion, is able to adapt himself to the various shades of temperament and character, and the opposite of disappointment, which is bliss, fills his soul.

And if the free-souled man meets apparent reverses, if his lady love throws obstructions in his way, in order to test his temper, he will not be disappointed, but will welcome each rebuff as a means by which to prove to her his desirability. He could not do this if his unconscious passion were fixated upon his mother imago. If it is thus fixated, he is always looking, unconsciously, for a mother, and is bound to be disappointed, and particularly by a wholesome woman, as she is looking, unconsciously, too, it may be, for a man and not for a child.

The man with the liberated unconscious passion is the one who is able to achieve real happiness. The other is not. The one can adapt himself to the environment the woman supplies. The other cannot. The one is able to grow; the other has had his growth arrested. The one is able to mould his woman still closer to his heart's desire, because he has no false ideal to lose. The other has to struggle between shattering an extraneously imposed ideal and giving it up entirely.

Only the man with the liberated unconscious passion is really free to achieve a union with a woman well developed physically and mentally. It requires all the greatness of heart and mind to be able to give constantly of oneself, because of a confidence in the infinity of power. Fear, which haunts every step and emasculates every movement of the man enslaved by the mother imago, is unknown to the free man.

And he knows, too, that, if one woman fails

him, there are others. Not looking for one only woman, the replica of his mother imago, he can wait, too, until he is absolutely sure of the character of his beloved. The imago-slave has the childish trait of needing instant compliance and quick results. The imago-free is able to abstain from immediate gratification because his life is more expansive, and his goal more distant. He can really make a more complete marriage, because he can look at the proposition from every point of view, and not merely from the point of view of whether his intended wife in every respect fits his unconscious dummy—the imago— for he does not go around carrying this dummy in his soul, having cast it off at the time he dropped his toys and took up man's work.

G. A Peculiarity of the Love Instinct

Christianity took man out of the mire of lust coagulated of the débris of decadent Rome and made possible the love of man and woman as it never had been before. It exalted motherhood in the Madonna, and laid the basis for a new type of marriage in which true mutuality might continue, a basis however on which no very notable structure has been erected, as undoubting love has had to struggle with Roman imperial property legality on the one hand and asceticism on the other.

The incest barrier referred to in the preceding chapters is the unconscious impediment which Nature has put in the way of inbreeding, and which civilization has extended more or less to all expression of the love instinct. A comparison of the behaviour of the two main animal appetites, hunger and sex, reveals a curious peculiarity distinguishing man from other animals, and distinguishing man's love hunger from his food hunger, although the two cravings are biologically connected in ontogenetic development. Of all other animals except man it may be said that the food hunger is irregularly periodic, while the sex hunger is regularly periodic. In man the reverse seems to be the case. Barring the periodicity of menstruation, in which woman closely resembles the animal, there is no time nor season generally governing the expression of the human love instinct. The birth-rate varies slightly with the seasons in some countries, but not to the extent that the animal birth-rate is regulated.

Furthermore man's love hunger differs from his food hunger in the fact that he never has to use abstinence or variety to whet his appetite for food, nor does he have to resort to mental procedures to give piquancy to his food in order to increase his appetite. One becomes habituated to a certain food and does not feel compelled to change, in order to gain satisfaction from eating. While the mental element does indeed enter, to a certain degree, it is not the controlling element. Foods well cooked and elegantly served are more enjoyable, but even badly cooked and served foods still satisfy and nourish. If food were absolutely free, people would still enjoy it just as much.

It is markedly different with the love instinct, which requires an obstruction in order to mount to the loftiest expression. " In times when the satisfaction of love found no difficulties, as occasionally during the fall of ancient civilizations, love became worthless and life empty; and there was necessary a strong reactionary influence to restore the indispensable emotional values." " The psychical value of the need for love falls, as soon as its satisfaction is made easy. An obstruction is needed to force the libido upward, and, where the natural obstructions to satisfaction do not apply, men have at all times inserted them, in order to be able to enjoy love." *

It thus appears that there is something in the nature of the love instinct that makes it in a sense inconsistent with itself. It may be due, as has been suggested, to the anatomy and physiology of the reproductive processes themselves. Or it may be due to the fact that in humans so

* Freud, *l. c.*, page 48.

much of the mental processes has become involved. Conscious mental association has linked so many human activities with the love instinct that, for the transference of both conscious and unconscious passion, permanently to one mate, a very elaborate system of mental activities is necessary.

Another peculiarity of human love hunger is not alone its ontogenetic connection with food hunger, but its derivation from, or synthesis out of, so many separate elements, over-emphasis on any one of which in one partner may make difficult the transfer of conscious and unconscious passion in both ways. A man for whom the love act reaches its consummation in mere cutaneous contact, or a woman for whom the masochistic component requires a certain amount of physical pain, are both examples of the over-emphasis in adult years of an essentially infantile component, and can never become happily mated.

These are extreme cases, to be sure; but the multitudinous love specifications, the more numerous the higher the civilization, are so assorted that the chances of a perfect transfer are less and less,—without natural insight and adaptability, or without the help of a psychological analysis of the emotions. I have indicated in the preceding chapters one of the principal impediments to a complete transfer—the parent imago. In a subsequent volume I shall hope to take up the various combinations of conscious and unconscious passion and insight without regard to the composite nature of the love instinct itself.

It might be advantageous here, however, to discuss somewhat more in detail the elements out of which real adult love is an organic synthesis.

H. *Elements Synthetized in Love*

1. Muscle Instinct

'As there are from fourteen to sixteen years of the child's life during which physical growth is the most notable accomplishment of the individual, it would not be surprising if the muscular development resulted in a tendency to get satisfactions out of the mere use of the muscles. 'All children gain a great satisfaction from this, normally; and, if the satisfactions thus gained remained the primary satisfactions of the individual, he or she would continue to be emotionally a child. Great athletes, and all those whose chief interest is in physical exertion without creative result, such as the production of something of social value, some effect other than the raising of a record, which is but the comparison of their own physique with that of others—all such people are primarily grown-up children, and their loves are likely to be autoerotic in other respects as well. The muscle instinct is of course a necessary element in the development of the psyche, but, like all other instincts, it may preponderate in such a way as to destroy the balance of an otherwise proportioned development. Mrs. Evans, in her book previously mentioned, has given a very instructive example of a boy who suffered, and whose family suffered, from the over-development of his muscle instinct.

Very early in childhood a pleasure is experienced from the mere contraction of all the muscles of the body, and with it is associated the sense of power, a source of infinite satisfaction. This sense of power is felt notably upon the perception by the child of its effect on some other person, animal or thing. Squeezing other children or animals or tearing things apart gives the normal child a perfectly normal pleasure, which is inevitably associated in its mind with pain or expression of pain on the part of human or animal object of its strength; so that the pleasure is at least partly attributed to the pain inflicted upon the other. No one who has carefully observed children teasing and mauling each other will fail to note the pleasure gained by the very act of inflicting pain, and that this pleasure is very intense. The greater the outcries and struggles, the keener the enjoyment. Parents naturally attempt to restrain this tendency to get great pleasure out of pain inflicted by the child upon some other child or upon some animal, partly because of some possible retaliatory injury, possibly because of the adults' superior sympathy for the victim.

2. Sadism-Masochism

But however strongly developed, or however forcefully repressed by external influences, this trend of the natural child personality, which is called Sadism, is an always to be expected trait in all children. As it is indissolubly linked by frequent experiences with satisfactions of an exceedingly high degree, it is inevitably associated with all pleasure, and as an independent element, leads, in its extreme form, to murder. The ecstatic pleasure of the individual who has "killed his man" is well known and has been described by some writers. Sadism is thus an independent element in the love emotion, containing, as it does, the factor of aggrandizement of the ego, from which is derived a fundamental and perennial satisfaction.

Sadism is called a partial trend of the libido, because it is always accompanied by a corresponding or balancing antagonistic trend, to

which has been given the name Masochism. This
is a pleasure indissolubly linked with the expression of power, but with that of the exertion of
power over oneself by some other person. It
will be seen at once that Masochism is a trend
that is, on the average, more developed in women
than in men, while Sadism is expected to have
a more or less prominent place in the man's
psychic make-up. Without a certain amount of
Sadism, no man could vanquish a rival in any
contest, because the pleasure of victory comes
alone from the sadistic trend and the satisfactions that it supplies.

Both Sadism and Masochism are present in
every individual man and woman, but in varied
proportions. Wherever a person's external acts
can be called sadistic, domineering, aggressive,
self-assertive, they are conscious compensations
for his repressed Masochism, and wherever his
acts can be called masochistic, self-abnegating,
self-sacrificing, altruistic, they are conscious compensations for repressed Sadism. When the
child is too well trained in unselfishness, he
becomes consciously masochistic in tendency and
is most likely as a grown-up individual later
to give many manifestations of his repressed
Sadism. One of these is an intense interest in
societies for the prevention of cruelty to children
or animals, activities which the individual gen-

erally does not associate with their true cause, the repressed Sadism.*

Both Sadism and Masochism are components of the love instinct, the former slightly more in evidence in the conscious life of man, the latter in that of woman. But each amount appearing in consciousness compensates for a corresponding amount in inverse proportion of the other in the unconscious of the individual. The more Masochism *appearing,* the more Sadism repressed, and vice versa. Both give pleasure, both cause satisfaction feelings. If external influences repress the aggressive component, the satisfaction is immediately secured by the other. The beggar exhibits his afflictions. A virtue is always made of necessity.

This comes from the fact that satisfaction (literally = Latin for *doing enough*) is the result of a relaxation of a tension of a group of muscles, either great or small muscles, either voluntary or involuntary, either conscious or unconscious. Unconscious satisfactions come from conscious strains. The satisfaction of consciousness itself is always and continuously the result of strains, most of which are unconscious. In other words, life is a rhythm of tensions and relaxations, harmonious or otherwise, of muscles

* See Wilfrid Lay: *The Child's Unconscious Mind,* N. Y., 1919, p. 143.

of one variety or another. The occurrence of this thought rather than another is the effect of the combined forces, one tending to keep it out of consciousness, the other to bring it in. Biologically the greatest tension is that tending to reproduction, and the greatest relaxation and therefore the greatest satisfaction is that of the relaxation of all the muscles great and small, and all the psychic tensions associated with it, concerned in the reproductive act. But as cowards die many times before their deaths, the tensions of all the groups of greater and smaller muscles used in carrying out the desires springing from the fundamental cravings of the individual, will periodically become automatically relaxed.

I. *Automatic Relaxation*

So universal is this that it may truly be said that in animals and humans, particularly young humans, but yet in many of greater age, all tensions are automatically relaxed. The satisfactions then secured, the feelings of satisfaction then experienced, are inevitably associated with the external sensations accompanying the relaxation. Many a person forces his will on another and explains or apologizes and is afterward forgiven.

The principle of universal relaxation of tension applies in every sphere of human thought and activity, and accounts for the phenomenon of Masochism, without which principle it would be hard to explain why any one should gain pleasure in painful circumstances. It is not literally true that they get satisfaction *out of* the pain itself, but every pain except the most excessive, containing actual destruction of tissue, is necessarily accompanied by a tension. The contortions of any child who has been hurt illustrate both the tension and the relaxation. And relaxation is satisfaction. It is the muscle's *doing enough,* and, when the enough has been reached, the feeling of satisfaction is present and is associated with the pain. The pain is then, by a universal rule of human thought, considered to be the cause of the pleasure. It certainly is not the cause, but so strong is the unconscious inference of *propter hoc* from *post hoc,* that 99 out of 100 people think in this manner.

To this is added a number of other circumstances, among them two that stand out prominently. First is the fact that many are praised for their ability to do difficult things and to endure pain. Second, the principle of identification which is universally operative in all human minds. The person who is injured always unconsciously identifies himself with the other who does the injury. The muscularly weak woman identifies herself with the strong man who forces her to do anything, and no matter what she is forced to do, and no matter how much she is consciously eloquent in disclaiming the least approbation of the man's self-assertive acts, she nevertheless unconsciously realizes his power, chiefly by means of her identifying herself with him. Thus alone can she justify to herself the relaxation which inevitably takes place within her psyche. For when, e.g. the boy has forced the girl to go along with him to take a walk, the idea, which is in both their minds is externalized for both of them. The walk is taken; the deed is done by both equally. Even if the girl has to be dragged all the way, she identifies herself with her tormentor's strength, possibly with the thought that she made him put forth that amount of strength, and possibly that she would have done the same if she had been a boy.

As has been indicated in another section, much relaxation and its accompanying satisfaction is experienced by people who merely see some others doing something that they would like to do themselves, e.g. play ball or act in a play, or do some deed of heroism. That this is so strong as to overcome even the fear of death was plentifully evidenced in the alacrity with which our young men went to war.

3. Exhibitionism

Two other partial trends, beside Sadism and Masochism, enter in as components of the love instinct, and are normally characteristic of all children, but in adults are repressed or sublimated. These, like the previously mentioned Sadism and Masochism, have, one an active, and the other a passive phase. The active one of these two partial trends is the tendency to get satisfaction linked up with looking or seeing or peeping, and the other with being looked at or being seen. It might be thought that the exhibitionist, in making a show of herself, is active, but this is not the case, because she gets no satisfaction unless she is looked at. She would not pose alone, except before a glass. Her pleasure comes from the active attention of other persons.

The feminine pronoun here suggests what is really the truth, namely, that the passive phase of this partial trend is more characteristic of women than of men. This is shown, as pointed out by Frink * even by the clothing of civilized men and women. Either the women expose more of their bodies, thus getting the satisfaction of this

* H. W. Frink: *Morbid Fears and Compulsions,* New York, 1918.

component of their unconscious love instinct, or
they wear clothing more colourful and appealing
to the eye, all with the unconscious purpose of
attracting toward themselves the activity of the
eyes of men. On the other hand men instinctively
care less to be looked at than to look. Man is the
discursive, errant, inventive, discovering sex.
His activity leads him to investigate not only
ocularly but with hands and with tools, to
poke, to pry, to penetrate into things perceptible
in order to discover the imperceptible lying behind them. In all of this he may also be satisfying the desires arising from his unconscious
sadistic trend. Biologically one might ask how
is the zoosperm to reach the secluded ovum except by means of much investigating and sadistic
activity?

These two double traits, Sadism-Masochism
and active and passive exhibitionism are apparently different, only because they are satisfactions associated with different spheres of sense.
Seeing and being seen, hearing and being heard,
smelling and being smelt, touching and being
touched, hurting and being hurt are all in parallel lines but at different ends. They go back
finally to a fundamental difference between acting and being acted upon, with each of which is
associated its peculiar satisfaction. That each
one of them contains a tension which must be

relaxed whatever happens has been already indicated.

4. Erogenous Zones

To these active-passive sources of satisfaction may be added the purely sensational (passive) ones of the so-called erogenous zones. These are parts of the body from which, in infancy and childhood come keen pleasures that are not normally retained into adulthood as prime sources of pleasure. In childhood any one of these regions of the body may be stimulated in its appropriate way and not invite the individual to further stimulation of other zones. The erogenous zones are usually considered to include the oral, anal and genital, with possibly others of wide extent, such as the cutaneous. It is conceived that any one of these, even the genital, may in infancy be stimulated independently, with approximately equal satisfaction and none of them constitute merely an approach to any other.

But the synthesis of these partial trends and erogenous zones into a unitary function, at or about the time of puberty, causes all the others to be subordinated to the genital zone, in such a way that any satisfaction or relaxation of tension in any one of them immediately causes a great tension in some one or others, and, finally, the main tension in the genital zone itself. It is as if in children no zone or partial trend necessarily affected any other, but in adults excitement in any one necessarily excited all the others and finally the genital.

In an automobile there is what is known as a firing order of the cylinders, and they are fired always in the same order which is never that of their position in the car. So it may well be that there is a sort of firing order in the erogenous zones and partial trends that is different for different people. The force of the explosions in all of the cylinders of an automobile is as nearly equal as engineering science can make it. In the amount of satisfaction gained by the adult from the different sources just mentioned, we do know that there is not a little variation, some of these erotic cylinders having much, and others little, power developed. In some individuals we know also that one or more of these cylinders has no compression, so to speak, or no spark, with the result that the car proceeds with a jerky motion. In the child, to carry out the internal combustion engine simile, there is never more than one cylinder operative at a time, the child being completely satisfied with one at a time, and switching off from one to another cylinder, whether he has two or twelve. The internal secretions at the time of puberty integrate and organize the various erogenous zones and the partial trends, just as a skilled mechanic can connect the cylinders with the proper wires and set the whole engine to fire in proper order of cylinders, and the full power of the individual is then capable ot development.

But it is obvious that any one of the satisfactions of the originally unsubordinated sources of pleasure, by being retained as a principal source in the final composition of the love instinct or unconscious passion, may result in an undesirable lack of integration of the passion. This is the real cause of the arrest of emotional development in the individual and prevents him or her from being truly adult, no matter how much grown up.

But even in the well-proportioned development of the adult love instinct out of the diverse factors of which it is composed, there is clearly visible the contradiction or antagonism between some of the elements. There is, for example, a striking opposition between on the one hand merely seeing and on the other receiving· sensations from other sense organs, external or internal; and an over-emphasis of visual enjoyment will tend, in some people at least to underrate the satisfactions derivable from other sensations or activities. Food hunger contains no such antagonisms. Love hunger is essentially full of innate oppositions. The visual appeal of the human form is not made equally by all parts of it, except possibly in persons aesthetically trained; nor is the tactual appeal of one person to another made equally by all parts to every other part.

Therefore it is a matter of the greatest importance to be able to analyze the emotions of love into their elements and to be able to detect those that are over-emphasized in the unconscious passion. The importance consists chiefly in this: that by bringing into consciousness, as we can indeed do, by the appropriate methods, what was formerly in the unconscious, we are able to correlate it with what is already in consciousness, or at any rate in the fore-conscious, and thereby gain an actual control over the forces in the unconscious mind—forces which are primal in their strength and unlimited in extent of time. The unsatisfied, unsuccessful, unhappy individual is he (or she) who is prevented by some repression from becoming aware of the undeveloped state of some one or more elements of the unconscious passion. An arrest of development here is inevitably going to cause a lack of growth in all the functions of body and mind derivable from this one element.

J. *Sublimation of the Elements*

It happens in all people that the primary satisfactions derived from the stimulation of the different erogenous zones may be given up, if some activity is pursued that gives an indirect satisfaction. It really gives the same satisfaction, but the action is different. For example, it is not socially approved in our present civilization for men and women to go barefooted, or to expose more than their hands and faces undraped. But a woman with beautiful feet and legs will derive conscious satisfaction from showing them to other people. If the feeling of satisfaction from showing her bare feet be very strong, it may still be a feeling in the unconscious. The majority of people cannot tell why they like to do various things. Some will generally say that they like to do this or that, but they cannot explain why. They get a feeling of satisfaction that is partly conscious, partly unconscious. The attempt to tell why one likes one kind of business rather than another, or one form of amusement rather than another, or foods or anything else, is always subject to two impediments.

1. Many people consider the question why they prefer tennis to golf, or athletics to reading, or any such question, as a challenge imply-

ing the disagreement or criticism of the questioner. This immediately arouses all the innate antagonism of the person being questioned, and he endeavours by any means whatsoever, logical or otherwise, to justify his preference, falling into the universal error of rationalization, i.e. assigning conscious reasons for unconsciously determined actions. 2. The cause being at least partly in the unconscious, only a person who has been analyzed or has succeeded in partly analyzing himself, can give a complete account of the cause of any of his acts. Primarily they are all caused by the unconscious craving for self-preservation or race preservation. The satisfaction feeling derived from doing a good job of plumbing will be partly determined by the satisfaction associated with the stimulation of one of the erogenous zones, and only partly from the later acquired association of satisfaction with approval of others, with money well earned, with muscles reasonably fatigued, etc.

Similarly the satisfaction from dancing barefooted on the stage will be partly conditioned by the gratification of exhibitionism, one of the components of later love instinct, and partly by the fact that others approve and applaud the performance, that the performance has been studied and arranged with great care, and with a view to light, colour, grace of motion and analogy with the moods or concepts of the piece of literature or music represented by the dance. There cannot be the slightest ethical objection made reasonably by the most prudish critic of the performance, if the exhibition of the undraped foot is not the sole object aimed at by the performer. Direct exhibitionism is a crime punishable by law. Indirect exhibitionism is not only not a crime but it is a beneficial act in that it enables the observer to look at nature through the eyes of humanity. It informs flesh with love, because love is the activity that transforms the material into the spiritual. It is the psychic element itself, in a world of physical matter. Indirect exhibitionism is the satisfaction of merely showing a part of the body, or even a concept of the mind, when this showing is combined with the satisfaction of contributing to the welfare of other people, either through their entertainment, their support, or their further development along physical or psychical lines. The person who can add to the joy or success of other humans, even by the artistic unveiling of any part of the body, or the action of any part of the unveiled body, is a valued member of society, and is doing his or her part in helping society to do what it wishes to do, which is to develop as an ever-growing organic unity.

I wish it could be said so clearly that no one

would fail to understand it, that not only is there no obloquy attachable to the various indirect exhibitionisms active or passive, but the very fact of their being indirect is the result of directed thinking and not of phantasying, and is therefore on the path toward scientific accomplishment and away from mere autoerotic thinking. One person of the opposite sex may be hugely entertaining by direct exhibitionism, but it takes much careful thinking to arrange any degree of entertainment for more than one person. The complications entering into the total situation where more than one are to be entertained are such that success in this undertaking requires the expenditure of a large amount of psychic energy on things distinctly *not* exhibitionistic. Thus is fulfilled the destiny of life to vivify more and more of inanimate nature.

The difference between a thousand men and women looking at semi-draped actors and actresses on a stage, and thirty men and women making pictures in charcoal or in oil colours of a nude model is only that there is predominant an indirect *passive* exhibition in the theatre, and indirect *active* exhibition in the art school. The difference in degree of nudity does not affect the matter. The actors are passive exhibitionists, their exhibitionistic element being reduced to a minimum, the audience are active exhibitionists (voyeurs) with the exhibitionistic element similarly somewhat reduced, but of the four groups concerned they are the least creative. The nude model is a passive exhibitionist, but her function in the community is of recognized value, and she does not pose for only the gratification of being looked at. She does it sometimes unwillingly, to be sure, as far as her own conscious life goes, however much unconscious gratification she may get. The students are active exhibitionists but of the most indirect variety possible, as their efforts are directed solely to representing the model in an extremely complicated medium, which so engrosses their minds that any thought of prudery is absolutely excluded. Their satisfactions are gained primarily through the activities of their hands and brushes and the elaborate technique connected with them.

This illustrates very well the network of motives that may be found in every human activity, and shows how clearly a person is either unwilling or unable to tell why he gets satisfaction out of any special activity. For no one will be able to deny that the actor gets a small part of his satisfaction out of passive exhibitionism, or that the audience get a large part of theirs out of actively looking. The satisfaction feeling may be augmented by any or all of the elements of the total situation.

Finally it should be emphasized that not only is this kind of exhibitionism not a crime or a sin or even a fault, but it is a meritorious action in so far as it conduces toward the organized life of the social unit, which it can do in many ways. Even though they are only exhibited on board fences, attractive posters can help in stirring people to deeds of patriotism. It is not a shameful thing to trace, as the analysts do, the activities of men to one or more components of the love instinct, but on the contrary a noble deed to show people how their love instinct can be gratified in carrying on almost any kind of activity, provided only it has the aim of satisfying at the same time a number of people.

K. *Platonic Love*

Those who believe in love as the desire for the beauty that is above sense are either sublimating, or repressing into the unconscious, the desires for sensual gratification springing thence. Both of these have been recommended. The latter is fraught with danger. Only in case the unconscious passion has not been repressed but sublimated can its frank expression be checked without injury to the body, which contains the libido as a pipe contains steam under pressure.

In the cult of feminine beauty flourishing in the Renaissance and rationalized by means of Plato's dicta, we have the transmutation of a desire to touch into a desire to see. This implies only that the satisfaction gained by the gratification of the desire to touch is artificially replaced by the much more stimulated and dynamized natural satisfaction secured by sight. At that time the extraordinary development of pictorial art and of the characteristics of literary art which largely evoked visual images, showed how men's creative desires were shunted from reproductive creation, which in the preceding dark ages had become so animal as to have lost its human savour, to a productive creativeness. Then men began afresh to use their eyes. Things visible took on new meanings of other sense qualities. The ability to liken the things of vision to things of taste, smell, action and organic sense quality was the re-birth that then took place— the re-birth of a new vision, to which most aptly was given the name enlightenment.

The greatest literary work of art of that time, the *Divine Comedy,* is a visual dream. Into the visual form Dante put every detail of the philosophy and religion of his day, though some of the concepts of both religion and philosophy are almost incompatible with the visual form. His ecstatic vision is but an attempt to express in optical impressions the acme of love's consummation, an emotional state not biologically connected primarily with the sense of sight but with that of touch, and mediated through well-nigh unwordable organic sensations. It would take too much space to give a hundredth of the citations in which Dante's language shows an excessive over-valuation of the merely visual quality of consciousness.

Plato himself was a visualizer and his ideas are visions. The Platonic love of the Renaissance was the transmutation of the object of love into a thing to be seen and not touched, save possibly symbolically by means of the kiss. A tremendous importance was suddenly attributed to sight alone; the various visual qualities of line, form, hue and tint were invested with meanings that consisted in the images of the other sense qualities not previously associated with sight. For, as every one of the twenty-odd qualities distinguished by conscious attention may serve, each as a kind of meaning for each and every other one, it is possible for man so to associate these mental activities that all or many of them shall be related to one of them, for example, sight.

By this procedure the satisfaction derived from looking at a peach may be successfully substituted for that ordinarily derived from eating it, and a putative satisfaction may, by training, be ascribed to the sight of anything, whether or not' that thing naturally and instinctively had for humans the tendency to arouse satisfaction solely through its visual appeal. Thus not only can the feeling of satisfaction be drilled, in some regions of the mind, to march with vision instead of with touch, as has been Nature's custom for eons of evolution, but the satisfactions innately associated with every other sense quality can be detached from that quality and attached to different visual qualities. The ecstatic pleasure in motion, whose archetype is that of prenatal uterine cradling, a pleasure that children get in swinging and in sliding down hill, and " grown ups " in motoring, is disassociated from those activities and reassociated with the motion of the eye in following a curved line in a picture or a statue.

Platonic love is then in its highest expression, visual love—the training of the psyche to gain the same satisfactions from seeing as, in the average man and woman, are secured through all the other avenues of sense. As vision is the richest of the senses in permutations and combinations of qualities, it easily results, with the help of language, that abstractions are formed from visual sense qualitites; and then one hears of the love above sense, and one is told that by following the shadow (note the visual word) one may finally reach the source of light itself.

From the psychological point of view of modern analysis it must have already occurred to the reader that there is at least a slight analogy between Platonic love and the infantile exhibitionism already discussed. No matter how exalted and spiritual it may become, it is but an offshoot of the tree of life at a lower level on the elevation of development. Even so, it *may,* in some cases, be a perfectly socially available substitute for the fruitful love of perfect marriage.

Those who profess Platonic love should question themselves as to the true relations of their unconscious to their conscious passion. In most love of people of opposite sex for each other, even if the sensual or passionate current is not acknowledged to exist, it nevertheless does exist, but in the unconscious; and the manifestations of it into conscious thoughts and acts are not by the individual himself recognized for what they really are. But the existence of the passionate current may in some people be consciously recognized and may at the same time be drawn off in extra energy devoted to the elaborate praise of the visual beauty of the adored, or in sedulous repeated acts of devotion (copious source of satisfaction feeling) or even in the most extravagant lamentation at the cruelty of fate in not permitting the lovers fully to possess each other. Feeling demands action, and a deep desire for contact can be dissolved in a fierce effort of flight, either literal or symbolical.

The purely " Platonic " attachment of the man for another man's wife may be a salutary thing for both of them only if the unconscious passion of each is necessarily, because of some impossible circumstances, detached, by unkind fate, from the legitimate spouse. But if a man and wife are both married to each other, i.e. if both passions of each are transferred to the other, there will be no possibility in the case of either of them, of any attachment, whether called Platonic or otherwise, to any other person.

L. *The Rejuvenated Parent Imago*

The concept of the rejuvenated parent imago has been lately proposed. It is conceived that the mother or father imago in man or woman, instead of being so fixated as to be unchangeable, may yet determine the man's or woman's choice of a mate, and then become so flexible as to adapt itself to her as she really is, or to him as he really is, so that the transfer of unconscious passion to her or to him is perfect. Rejuvenation would then be the change from the inflexi-

bility of an early strong mother or father imago
to the accommodating adaptability of a man's
or woman's unconscious passion to the essential
attractiveness of a really desirable mate. And
we can conceive that if the impressions made
on the man by the woman were sufficiently
pleasurable, they would altogether obliterate
any unpleasant ones coming from her not corresponding, in this or that minor respect, with
the imago. And everything would go on well
enough until the points of difference, from which
the man gets no unconscious gratification of his
unconscious desires, are more numerous than the
points of resemblance.

This is the more plausible from the fact that
the parent imago in many people is a forma-
tion not in the lowest depths of the unconscious,
where there is almost utter formlessness, but in
its upper strata or even in the fore-conscious itself. Indeed the lowest depths of the unconscious
may be said to be blind and altogether insentient
specifically, so that no discrimination between
women, or even between sexes, is possible; as if
only warmth, excitement and secretion were all-
sufficient. Also most inhibitions upon the gratification of the desires of unconscious passion
originate in the more conscious rather than in
the less, and what they inhibit is the actions
which would have been carried out in the line

of fulfilling the fundamental unconscious wishes. Nature abhors a vacuum, but only up to certain limits (below thirty-two feet of water, for example) and instinct abhors incest, but only in the upper, and not in the lower levels of the unconscious.

There is thus an antagonism always between the two extremes of consciousness and the unconscious, the lowest strata of the latter ever craving expression in any and every activity, particularly those affording pleasurable sensations, and the extreme of consciousness always discriminating between degrees of desirability, and repressing the activity suggested by the lowest strata, and encouraging and furthering activities which will fit into a form impressed upon amorphous desire by upper levels of mentality.

The antagonism is analogous to that of the many pairs of antagonistic muscles in the body, through whose action we stand or sit or walk or run. Just as a specific posture is maintained in the body, so is a definite wish formed in the mind, by the ambivalence of contrary tendencies, the stronger always giving the direction. Those suffering from serious mental disorders are merely examples of the inability of the conscious and modern inhibition to overcome the unconscious and archaic desire, so that the latter is outwardly manifested, whereas, in all so-called normal people, the Paleozic cravings are present, but are controlled from above, or, if not from the highest conscious levels, at any rate from those above the ones whence emanate the oldest and simplest desires. Any one who kisses a horse or a dog or in any way caresses an animal is satisfying an archaic, unconscious desire for warm, soft contrectation, but one which has not been inhibited by society, that is, by the requirements of society that have entered the consciousness of the person in question.

So that it is quite possible to have a parent imago rejuvenated, and still remain a comparatively faithful imago, provided the conscious life of both partners has been such as to allow the one to do all the adapting, in case the other's imago is firmly fixed, or, vice versa, to allow the other to adapt completely to the one, in case this one's is the fixed imago. But, if both are fixed and neither can do any adapting, the result is hopeless, unless analytical psychology can be resorted to, for the purpose of teaching either or both of them how to make the necessary adaptations.

This fixity of the imago is a moot point in psychiatry. No one is absolutely certain that any person's psyche is thus rigid, because it can never be positively stated that every effort has been made to make it malleable. Heavy enough sledge-hammer blows will change the shape of almost any metal, but if the soul be crystallized, into a rock, the blows of the environment will have no effect on it, if they be light, but if they be heavy, they will crush it. We have always to take into consideration the relation between environmental pressure and innate consistency of soul, if we may be allowed the phrase. It seems quite permissible, in view of William James' division of people into tender minded and tough minded.

M. *Homosexuality*

This so-called perversity is merely a recrudescence of the desires for contact and warmth, emanating from the lowest strata of unconscious craving. A type of people called " urnings " have been described by some psychologists. They are persons said to be women with masculine souls, or men with feminine souls. They exhibit inverse secondary psychic sexual tendencies, the women either forming more or less Platonic friendships with women or with very feminine men, and the men with mannish women or most masculine men. But the variations here are innumerable. The point to be noticed particularly is that the men exclusively fond of men's society and the women solely devoted to women's companionship are likely to have a psychical nature in which the more archaic desires crop out. These would naturally become bisexual in their actions, devoting their attention equally to men and women (and there are some such), were it not for the fact that conventionality makes it easier for men to form intimate relations with men, and women with women, than for men and women together. And in social or economic groups of men such as armies, there is an added facility of all kinds of intercourse, the extreme of which leads to homo-sexual practices.

That the conventions of modern society should thus lead to perversities is due, as are other evils, to society's present infantile state. In the evolution of social life, we have as yet reached only the childhood of the race. All our large community reactions are characterized by lack of insight and downright puerility. Democracy would be a perfect form of government, if the average intelligence age were three years older than its present age, which is about thirteen, and if the emotion age were that of the adult, instead of the infant or adolescent. There is no method of raising the first (the intelligence age) except that of the most intensive popular education, or of raising the second (the emotion age) except that of the most widespread enlightenment on matters of sexual psychology, which has as yet only "scratched the surface" and will be able to penetrate into the most intimate relations of humanity only after long and painstaking efforts.

The fixity of the parent imago itself is an arrest in the development of the psyche from infancy to adulthood. If the innate neural disposition of the individual is reasonably elastic, he will be able to adapt himself to external circumstances in all respects, including his love life, although he may be otherwise and independently of his own disposition prevented from adapting, because of the wrong character of the environment. The environment of any child is wrong, if it contains to little or too much parental influence. Children have to begin quite early to have adventures in the world outside the family, and, if the parents are over particular or squeamish or dictatorial or themselves too crystallized, the effect on the child of either sex will be very harmful.

But in families with many children, the parent influence is spread thinner, and does not blight the young life, as a huge tree shades a sapling, taking the sunlight away from it. Not having so strong a parent imago, the boy or girl does not form such elaborate specifications about what a mate must have, and is more likely to adapt to the mate bestowed by fortune than are those whose minds are too definitely made up by long and close association with inelastic adults.

Children so brought up have, formed in their souls, a parent imago that is capable of rejuvenation, because of the comparative elasticity and indefiniteness of its outlines. In them the parent imago is negligible in its effect, because it does not interfere with the transfer of unconscious passion. The majority of average happy marriages are between people of this type. We may almost say that an elastic and easily rejuvenated parent imago is a help, as it enables the young people to transfer to each other a large amount of affection, which, though it is of small account in the transfer of unconscious passion, is useful in making pleasant the external relations of married life.

With the absolutely happy married people I have no present concern, because they need no help, and sometimes no further insight. All others, however, may be aided in analyzing their troubles by a careful study of the elements of conscious and unconscious passion, here presented, and the combinations of these elements, with and without insight. The analysis needs patience and restraint and avoidance of hasty conclusions. But, for any man who has realized through self-analysis that his actions toward his wife are dominated by a mother imago, and are therefore essentially puerile, it should be quite possible to change his behaviour, particularly when he has realized that a childish behaviour not only repels the unconscious passion of his wife, but tends thereby to render her old and unattractive before her time, while those whose unconscious passion is given legitimate expression, remain young and attractive indefinitely. And when the woman realizes that only by the complete transfer of passion, both conscious and unconscious, to her husband, can she prevent him from being an inevitable unconscious bigamist, and cause a conflict in his soul, which actually divides it against itself, and makes him lack unity in all the battles of life, she will give her best thought to self-analysis to the end of understanding herself better and promoting the mutual understanding of herself and her husband and the health and happiness of both.

Those intending to marry are not less but more concerned in the matters taken up in this volume, for their future happiness depends on a wise choice of life partner, and the actions, before close acquaintance has ripened into conscious passion, should be clearly indicative of the unconscious trends. There is still opportunity for such people to study themselves, and acknowledge frankly to themselves and to each other, if they find that indications show their unconscious passion is not enlisted. They should enlarge their acquaintance, and gain a greater chance of being happy. And if, on self-examination, they find that they have absolutely no conscious or unconscious inhibitions against each other, they should not delay marriage, for the longer it is delayed, the more difficult it is to adapt each to other.

N. *Conscious Control*

Activities which originate in conscious life do reshape and redirect those of the fore-conscious, which in turn have an effect upon the activities of the lower, if not the lowest, strata of the otherwise unalterable unconscious. In this way indeed a conscious passion may finally overcome a previous infantile fixation of the unconscious passion upon the parent imago, and in this way both sublimations and repressions are effected. The unconscious passion of the boy for his mother is repressed, and desires for certain other kinds of activities are repressed, by this power of the verbal integration to inhibit the action.

Where the unconscious passion of the boy for the mother person is properly handled from the first, there is no such integration of fore-conscious mental activity necessary; it does not take place and, other things being equal, no fixation upon the mother imago occurs. If the inhibitory statements and actions of the mother person are no stronger than to impress merely the fore-conscious levels of the boy, whatever fixations are caused, whatever integrations take place, are not so deeply impressed as to give an actual and permanent shape, so to speak, to the unconscious levels themselves. There is many a youth fond of his mother whose unconscious passion has not been too deeply fixated. If this were not the case, the fruitful sexual relations would be mostly outside of the married state, and most of the children born would be called illegitimate.

And in all this we have to remember that the depth of the impression constituting a controlling mother imago is dependent upon two variable factors, the innate impressionability of the individual boy and the strength of the impression made. Some will be deeply impressed by a little, others not at all by much. Only those who have been deeply impressed are going to be permanently affected. But these are much more numerous than one would ordinarily suppose. The prevalence of prostitution is the proof of this, because so many men are unable physicaly or psychically to get satisfaction in the legalized way.

That physical satisfaction may be derived from illicit practices will be maintained by some, but it has been the aim of this book to show that love is the highest and the only satisfaction attainable by and through human activity, and that only that activity which enlists the entire personality is worthy of being called by the name of love. The failure of any part of the organism to function with the rest of the organism produces a strain, or racking effect, which, though it may not enter consciousness at that time, or later, will certainly have an undesirable effect, both physical and psychical, upon the individual. The failure of the individual organism to function as a harmonious whole is nowhere so deplorable as in the most vital relations of marriage; and the effect of this failure to achieve unity is felt not alone by the individuals composing the pair, but by their children, their neighbours and their community.

It is increasingly clear from the researches into the unconscious mental life of men and women that both body and mind are most healthy, when there is no unconscious conflict. There is likely to be such a conflict where there is a large amount of mental activity confined in the unconscious, whether it be primitive activity seeking an outlet, which is more difficult to find, the more highly complicated society becomes, or whether it be repressed mentality that has been thrust aside by conscious volition. More and more do we need to release into the wholesome air of conscious life the cravings and desires indigenous to, and, from time to time in our lives, jammed back into, the unconscious. Indeed it may be safely said that unless men and women are actively occupied every minute of their waking day in productive work, they will not be really happy, and if they are not happy, the cause lies in their ignorance of the strong life and elemental struggles going on below the threshold of consciousness. If they would but dare to face these struggles, they might eventually restore peace and unity within their own souls, where peace and unity are most necessary.

It is one thing to know that the struggle is taking place, and another, to take a hand in it. Surely the best humans, most productive of what in the long run will be of greatest advantage to society and its progress, will be found among those who are willing to take a part in this fight; and it is the hope of the present writer that with this book he may help to reveal the main outlines of the conflict in many a life that appears to contain nothing worse than an undertone of dissatisfaction, and to encourage all such persons to persevere in the rational study of their own problems. Such problems can never be fully sensed until their unconscious element is realized, and can never be solved if no reckoning be made of this unconscious factor. Only by recog-

nizing it, can we say, in the words of Rabbi ben
Ezra:

Let us cry, "All good things
Are ours, nor soul helps flesh more, now, than flesh
  helps soul."

INDEX

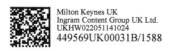

Milton Keynes UK
Ingram Content Group UK Ltd.
UKHW022051141024
449569UK00031B/1588

9 781138 875326